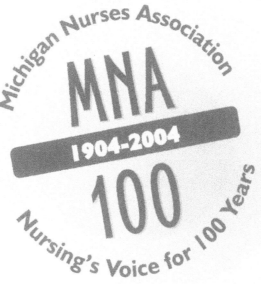

Michigan Nurses Association

MNA

1904-2004

100

Nursing's Voice for 100 Years

Proud of Our Past
Preparing for Our Future

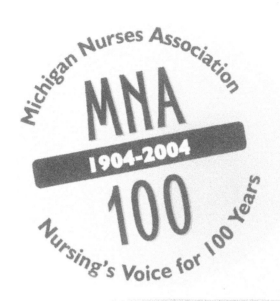

Proud of Our Past
Preparing for Our Future

A HISTORY OF THE
MICHIGAN NURSES ASSOCIATION
1904-2004

2310 JOLLY OAK ROAD • OKEMOS, MI 48864

888/MI-NURSE • www.minurses.org

Turner Publishing Company
Nashville, Tennessee

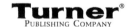

Turner®
PUBLISHING COMPANY

www.turnerpublishing.com

Library of Congress Control No. 2003107326

ISBN: 978-1-68162-252-1

R R H   0 9 8 7 6 5 4 3 2 1

Contents

Acknowledgements

The Centennial History of the Michigan Nurses Association was made possible by the efforts of many MNA members, staff, and friends, both past and present.

First and foremost, recognition goes to the following nurses who served on the Centennial Anniversary Steering Committee: co-chairs Marylee Pakieser & Mona White; Birthale Archie, Becky Baldwin, Vicki Boyce, Sue Brennan, Pam Chapman, Lynne Harris, Lola Johnson, Kathy Kacynski, Opal Lesse, Tara Nichols, and Jan Rosene. Special recognition goes to Birthale Archie who served as the Chief Coordinator and Editor of the history book as originally conceived, and was the driving force in making the book part of the centennial celebration plans.

The writing of this book was a collaborative effort under the direction of Carol Feuss, Director of Communication and Integrated Marketing. Additional staff compilation authors included: Ann Sincox, Editor and Writer, Jess Merrill, Projects and Special Events Director; and Tom Bissonnette, Executive Director. Layout and design of the book was done by MNA Graphic Designer, Lisa Gottlieb-Kinnaird.

Special thanks goes to Jan Coye, John Karebian, Jennifer Keenan, Joyce Losen, Toni Stevenson, Michelle Triantaflos, Pam Wojtowicz and the rest of the MNA staff who aided with typing, proof-reading, fact-checking, and/or photo-identifying and sorting.

The Michigan Nurse, dating back to 1928, was the primary source used to compile this history. Information from *The Michigan Nurse* was supplemented by documents from the State of Michigan Archives and personal histories. Thank you to the staff councils who included their histories and to Bette O'Connor-Rogers for coordinating this effort, to the many members who submitted their biographies to add richness to the history, and to the individuals who provided photos and other historical tidbits.

We also want to thank the Turner Publishing staff, who through their flexibility and professionalism enabled us to see this book to completion.

As with any book that tries to capture a history in too few pages, this contains only a small representation of our hundred year history. There are many stories that remain untold. And there are many stories yet to be written, as we anticipate our next hundred years.

The Centennial Steering Committee dedicates the MNA Centennial History Book to the memory of Mona White.

Introduction

In considering 100 years of the Michigan Nurses Association, I wondered, who were these nurses? Who did the work of the Association over the past century? What were their lives like and just what did they do as nurses? It's impossible to know from just looking at old pictures.

Recently, I had the opportunity to attend a tea to honor retired nurses in my home MNA chapter. A short biography was read for each nurse. As I listened to the varied backgrounds of each of these nurses, I realized that what these retired nurses have in common with those of us in nursing today is the caring we do for those around us. The caring is manifested in our work done in hospitals, clinics, schools, universities, local, state and national communities. We are real people, deeply involved and committed to making things better for ourselves and others.

As we move forward into our next 100 years, we should recognize and be thankful for the various backgrounds and talents that have contributed to where we are as the Michigan Nurses Association today. We should also recognize and be thankful for those who are busy moving the Association through today's challenges. This centennial history book of the Michigan Nurses Association provides that recognition and appreciation.

Even in the face of all of the differences among us, the common bond of trying to make things better and improve lives, binds us together. That is the bond that has sustained us, and I believe it is what will carry us through the next 100 years.

Cheryl Johnson, BSN, RN
MNA President

1904-1913

by Tom Bissonnette

Timeline

A State Association is Formed to Secure State Registration for Nurses

In the late 1800s and early 1900s, Americans were beginning to rid themselves of the belief that America should avoid getting involved with other countries' concerns. Because of its rapid economic and social growth, the United States had become a major world power. So when Cuban rebels began a violent revolution against Spanish rule in 1895, and a mysterious explosion sank the USS Maine in the Havana harbor, the US entered into what diplomat John Hay called "a splendid little war" with Spain. Although the Spanish-American war ended relatively soon, America had embarked on a course upon which it continues to this day. It is within this national context of leaving isolationism behind that the Michigan Nurses Association was born.

The Detroit Graduate Nurses' Association issued invitations to the graduate nurses of the State of Michigan to meet in Detroit on May 10, 1904, for the purpose of forming a State Association to secure State Registration for Nurses. What else was happening in 1904? Theodore Roosevelt was nominated without opposition at the Republican convention. He won easily over his opponent, Democrat Alton Parker of New York. Theodor Seuss Geisel (Dr. Seuss) was born, as were Archibald Leach (Cary Grant), Lucille Fay LeSueur (Joan Crawford), and Ladislav Loewenstein (Peter Lorre). Clara Barton, first president of the American Red Cross, resigned after holding the position for 23 years. Marie and Pierre Curie demonstrated that radium rays kill diseased cells.

About 100 graduate nurses, representing many hospitals and training schools throughout the state, and including nurses engaged in private duty nursing, responded to Detroit's invitation to meet. This excerpt from the April 1929 issue of *The Michigan Nurse* reflects the nurses' struggle for state registration.

Jessie Lennox, of Detroit, called the meeting to order, and Lystra E. Gretter was elected chairwoman. The Honorable W. H. Maybury gave the address of welcome. Dr. J. H. Carstens was present and on behalf of

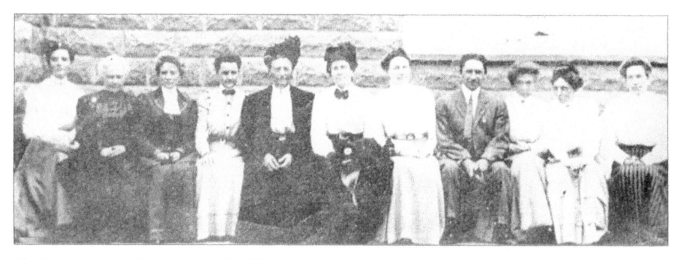

The Executive Board of 1909 meets in Grand Haven. Seated second from left is Linda Richards, America's first trained nurse; MSNA past presidents are Susan Fisher Apted (third from left), Anna Barbara Switzer (fifth from left) and Fantine Pemberton, seventh from left; Fred Schneider (eighth from left), represented Berrien County, and offered great assistance to MSNA in its efforts to secure registration for nurses.

the medical profession welcomed the visiting nurses. He gave a short account of the development and education of the trained nurse, and assured those present of the endorsement of the medical profession in the movement for State Registration. Judge C. A. Kent spoke on State Registration, giving valuable advice on framing a bill to present to the Legislature. He gave the plan cordial support, and encouragement. The object of the meeting was then stated by the chair. By a unanimous vote it was decided to form a State Association to effect State Registration for nurses.

A committee was appointed to register the delegates. Upon the presentation of their credentials and the payment of $1.00 they were admitted as members of the Michigan State Nurses Association [(MSNA), forerunner of the Michigan Nurses Association]. The committee previously appointed by the Detroit Graduate Nurses' Association to prepare a tentative draft of a constitution and bylaws presented its report, which was accepted. After careful reading as a whole and in seriatim*, and a full and free

*Seriatim means "in series"; apparently certain parts of the bylaws were questioned. Since General Henry M. Robert's *Pocket Manual of Rules of Order* had been in print since 1876, it's very possible the Association used what we now know as *Robert's Rules of Order* at that time.

discussion, it was, with two slight amendments, finally adopted.

The first annual meeting of the new Association was held in Grand Rapids in March, 1905, and at this meeting the first draft of the registration bill that had been prepared by Mr. Bryant Walker of Detroit, was presented.

Isabel McIsaac was a speaker at this meeting, and her subject was State Registration. Summarizing the history of the movement, she made a plea

Michigan State Nurses Association Board Members Elected 1904

President – Mrs. Lystra E. Gretter
First Vice-President – Miss Ida M. Barrett
Second Vice-President – Miss Ida Tracey
Recording Secretary – Miss Henrietta Potts
Corresponding Secretary – Miss Sarah Sly
Treasurer – Miss Mary C. Fletcher
Chairman Ways and Means Committee – Miss M. E. Smith
Chairman Nominating Committee – Miss Elizabeth L. Parker
Chairman Credentials Committee – Mrs. Lucia J. Lupinski
Chairman Arrangements Committee – Miss N. Ella Haight
Chairman Printing Committee – Miss Margaret Moore Ennis
Parliamentarian – Mrs. Emma A. Fox

for further educational advantages for nurses to elevate the standards of nursing schools.

The arguments and discussion about nurses' educational requirements for entry into practice continue in our present day.

The bill for State Registration of Nurses – Senate Bill 310 – was introduced by Senator Peeke of Jackson, on April 13, 1905. The only amendment made was that of a provision for the annual payment of $1.00 by every nurse for renewal of her registration, thereby ensuring enough money in the special fund to meet the expenses of the Board of Registration. The bill passed the Senate by unanimous vote on April 26th, but was defeated in the House because of its objection to the creation of another State Board.

Michigan's government defeated several similar bills for other health care professionals in the 1990s for the same reason: not wanting to create another State Board.

Far from being discouraged, renewed efforts were made through the Association's able legislative committee, of which Elizabeth Parker was the chairwoman, and with the cooperation of the

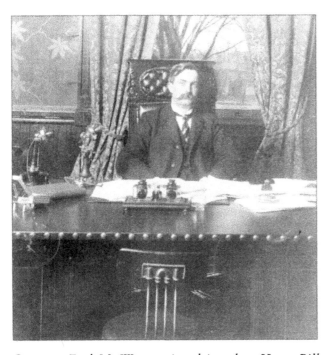

Governor Fred M. Warner signed into law House Bill No. 180, which created state registration for nurses.

nurses throughout the state to make a success of the second adventure. A legislative fund was created by individual contributions. Considerable time and energy were expended in the endeavor to enlist the understanding and support of legislators by the personal appeals of nurse residents in their respective districts. Promises of endorsement were secured from members of the medical profession. Prospects seemed favorable when on January 22, 1907, House Bill No. 89 was introduced through the House Public Health Committee by Representative George Lord.

The disconcerting discovery was made that an opposition bill, framed by the same physician who had pledged his aid to the nurses' bill, was likewise presented to the House by Representative Kelly. That bill was designed to assign the responsibility of the control of nursing standards and nurses' examinations, to the Board of Registration of Medicine. Both bills failed to pass.

Two more years of strenuous effort were required before the goal of State Registration was reached. House Bill No. 180, sponsored by Rep. Nelson C. Rice of St. Joseph, received 67 affirmative votes out of 74. It was rescued from burial in the Senate Public Health Committee by Senator Barnaby of Grand Rapids, who, ten minutes before the close of the session, moved that it be reported out for a vote. It was passed without a dissenting vote, was duly signed by Governor Fred M. Warner, and became a law.

One of the compromises that had been required of the nurses was the bill amendment that required the Registration Board to include one physician as well as the secretary of the State Board of Health, instead of having the Board comprised entirely of nurses.

Upon occasion, our modern Board of Nursing has had the Governor's office attempt to appoint, or actually appoint, a physician to one of the public member

Early Nursing Leaders in Michigan

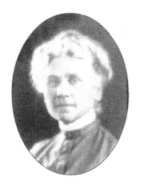

Lystra Gretter
First President – MSNA

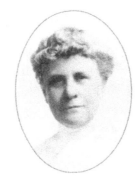

Elisabeth G. Flaws
Michigan's First Registered Nurse

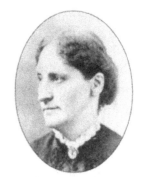

Linda Richards
America's First Trained Nurse

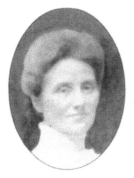

Mary Welsh
Counselor – MSNA

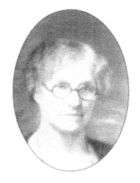

Mary Staines Foy
"Dean of Battle Creek Nurses"

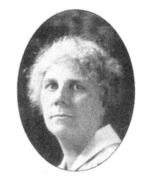

Henrietta Potts
Journal Committee – MSNA

positions on the Board of Nursing, although no current Board position is reserved for medicine.

The very first registered nurse in the State of Michigan was Elisabeth G. Flaws, then superintendent of Butterworth Hospital in Grand Rapids. She also served as the director of Butterworth's school of nursing. Her reputation throughout the state was so strong that she became not only a member of the first State Board of Registration of Nurses; she was elected the first president of the Board. There was one problem, however; Flaws wasn't registered! So, in the spring of 1910, she provided her credentials and was registered under the new law. Flaws had been a member of MSNA since 1905 and had worked diligently with the group to help secure the new law. Flaws was a native of Guelph, Ontario and had graduated from the Toronto General Hospital School of Nursing.

In this early period the Association numbered among its presidents our foundress, Lystra Gretter of Detroit, as well as Sarah Sly of Birmingham, Elizabeth Parker of Lansing, Anna Barbara Switzer of Ludington, Susan Fisher Apted of Grand Rapids, and Fantine Pemberton of Ann Arbor. These presidential pioneers, together with their able and loyal associates laid a strong foundation for the Association that is still being added upon today by their successors.

Michigan had the distinction of Linda Richards being a resident while she was organizing the school of nursing in the State Hospital in Kalamazoo. She and Isabel McIsaac contributed valuable service to the Michigan State Nurses' Association, and both were made honorary members. Many other leaders in the nursing profession responded at various times to invitations for their personal presence, and provided inspiring counsel on subjects that engaged the thoughtful interest of the Association members. Sophia F. Palmer helped immeasurably in the crusade for state registration; Katherine DeWitt gave enlightenment on private duty opportunities and responsibilities; Edna D. Foley brought expert judgment on tuberculosis nursing and Julia C. Stimson on social service. Eleanor Thompson presented a review of the field of mental hygiene nursing with a perspective of its infinite future possibilities. Mary C. Wheeler gave an address based on her experience as a member of the Illinois State Board of Examiners and Training School Inspector, and Harriet Leete provided insight and education on child welfare during this first decade of the Association's existence. Nursing the insane was a subject presented by Jennie Leece, of the Newberry State Hospital, from the expert knowledge she had gained by her training and experience.

Michigan contributed leadership and service to the national nursing organizations during these early years, a tradition that continues to this day, and records Sarah E. Sly as President of the

American Nurses' Association, Lystra E. Gretter as President of the National League of Nursing Education, and Agnes Deans as Secretary of the American Nurses' Association. Mary Staines Foy is closely associated with the early history of the Michigan State Nurses Association, and the standards which she maintained for nurses at the Battle Creek Sanitarium School of Nursing, and her contributions to nurse organization were outstanding.

Lucia J. Lupinski of Grand Rapids was the nurse chosen to represent the Association at the International Congress for the Study and Prevention of Tuberculosis in Washington in 1908. In the Michigan exhibit, which was in the charge of Dr. Warthin of Ann Arbor, a conspicuous place was given to a framed letter from

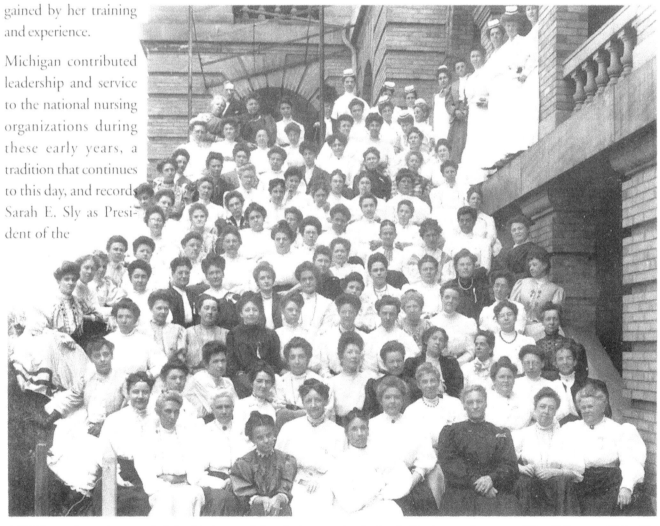

MSNA members who attended the third annual Association meeting in Battle Creek were the guests of Dr. Kellogg and Mrs. Foy at the Battle Creek Sanitarium. It was a rare event with a cordial welcome and perfect plans perfectly executed for the comfort, pleasure, and education of the guests.

the Association, expressing its interest, with the enclosure of a check for $15.00 to emphasize the good wishes for the success of the exhibit. Dr. Warthin stated that it was the first contribution he had received.

The Michigan nurses were hostesses to the American Nurses' Association in June, 1906. Isabel Hunter Robb, Lavinia L. Dock, M.E.P. Davis, and many other notable nurses were guests.

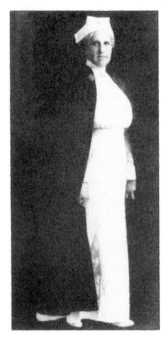

Jane A. Delano, founder of the Red Cross, spoke at MSNA's annual meeting in 1910.

From its earliest years the Michigan State Nurses Association assumed a share in the responsibilities of the Red Cross. The State and Local Committees on Red Cross Nursing Service functioned actively. The enrolled nurses had their loyalty and efficiency tested and proved in war, and in disaster relief. Jane A. Delano honored the Association with a visit on June 28, 1910, on the occasion of the annual meeting in Port Huron. She was on her way to the Philippines and made only a brief address, but those who were privileged to have contact with her radiant personality and to hear her inspiring words that conveyed the very spirit of the Red Cross, prized their memory of her visit. Elsbeth Vaughan was a Michigan nurse whose services to the Red Cross were outstanding.

In May, 1906, the Association was accepted into membership of the Michigan Federation of Women's Clubs, and it identified itself with many of the progressive movements the Federation sponsored. The report of Elizabeth Flans as a delegate to the annual convention in 1909, recommended that the Association instruct its delegate at the next meeting of the Federation to vote in favor of the constitutional amendment for woman suffrage.

A particularly impressive address on "Public Health Problems" was given by Linda Richards at the fourth annual Association meeting in Ann Arbor. She stressed prevention in health education, and it seems fitting here to quote her closing words: "We are a strong body of women, and with united effort we can accomplish much. We have a good record to look back upon, and you younger nurses have a glorious future to look forward to."

Those Who Marched

Lystra E. Gretter, RN (1858-1951)

By Elizabeth J. Miller, BSN, MSN, MPH, ABD

Lystra Gretter was an early national nursing leader who lived and worked the entire duration of her remarkable career in the metropolitan Detroit area, from 1889 through 1951. She was a contemporary of Lillian Wald and Jane Addams and had achievements in nursing, public health, and social welfare activities.

Born Lystra Eggert in Bayfield, Ontario, Canada in 1858, of Swiss and Dutch parents, she became American through naturalization. Her father, a surgeon in the Federal Army during the Civil War, moved the family to Greensboro, North

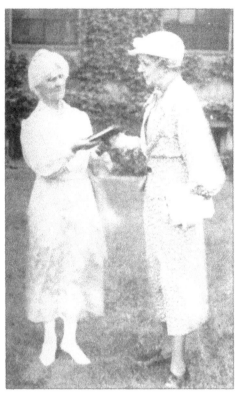

*Lystra E. Gretter (l) receives a copy of **The History of the Farrand Training School for Nurses** from co-author Agnes G. Deans.*

Carolina where Lystra spent her adolescent years being educated in private schools. She was married at age nineteen in North Carolina, and widowed with a three year old daughter at age twenty-six. Ms. Gretter made the decision to enter the Buffalo General Hospital Training School for Nurses in 1886. Upon completion of her nursing education in 1889, she became Principal (Superintendent) of the Farrand Training School for Nurses at Harper Hospital in Detroit (1889-1907). Within five years of her arrival at the School, Ms. Gretter initiated numerous educational reforms including reduction of students' workday to 8 hours a day instead of 12-15 hours; hiring of graduate nurses to function

as head nurses of hospital units instead of students; formulating a written text for nursing lectures (no books existed prior); and instituting regular planned course work for students.

Ms. Gretter was a founding member of the American Society of Superintendents of (Nursing) Training Schools (1893), which became the National League of Nursing. She began the Alumnae Associations in 1894, which was the forerunner of the Michigan State Nurses Association (us!). She was the prime mover to secure required state registration for registered nurses, being successful in doing so in 1909.

Ms. Gretter's most noteworthy work, however, could arguably have been her long-lasting efforts with the Metropolitan Detroit Visiting Nurses Association (Director, 1908-1923; Counselor Emeritus, 1923-1951). She had been a member of the VNA Board of Directors from its inception in 1898 and continued on with the Board until the late 1940s. In her drive to provide district home nursing care to the sick poor and to provide health teaching to the thousands of working-class immigrant families that were streaming into Detroit, Ms. Gretter set up innovative projects, proved their effectiveness, and then turned them over to a grateful Detroit Health Department to continue. These programs included the first health inspections of school children, the initial care and follow-up of the dreaded tuberculosis cases, and newly established mother/infant care clinics in Detroit.

Known as the "Dean of Michigan Nurses," Ms. Gretter also authored "The Florence Nightingale Pledge for Nurses" (1893), which was administered at all nursing schools from the time of its writing through the 1970s. She was a prime mover for the establishment of Chair of Public Health Nursing, at the University of Michigan (est. 1917), the first in the State. Ms. Gretter was known to her nursing colleagues throughout the state and nation as a progressive, energetic, persuasive public health leader who viewed health promotion and a positive overall environment as being necessary for the well-being of the general population.

Lystra Gretter was described by one of her contemporaries, a nurse colleague only known by the initials A.G.D., in the following excerpt: "She is a woman of extreme modesty, the embodiment of graciousness with a magnanimity of soul, a serene confidence in her associates, having the patience which is born of the union of knowledge and faith with the love of justice as a working principle for society. Ever a devotee of the 'great out of doors,' she spends her vacations in the country with her two grandchildren, who are her joy and delight."

Fifth District of the Michigan State Nurses Association Early Years 1904-1918

By Patricia Underwood, PhD, RN

Formation and Membership

The Graduate Nurses Association of Kalamazoo held its first meeting in 1904, the same year that saw the start of the Michigan State Nurses Association. On January 29, 1904, five nurses (Jessie Hewson, Minnie Johnstone, Florence Lee, Effie Pierce, and Elizabeth Pyle) attended the organizing meeting held in the home of Miss Effie Pierce who became the first president. The expressed purposes of this society were to:

1. "promote fellowship among its members,

2. advance the science of nursing, and

3. elevate the standards of nursing within its bounds" (minutes of the GNAK, January 29, 1904).

Over the course of the next few meetings a constitution and bylaws were drafted and approved by 13 charter members. Membership in the GNAK was open to any "graduate of a recognized training school" (Article II, Section I By Laws, 1904). The procedure for membership required interested nurses to be recommended by a GNAK member and have their credentials reviewed by the Board of Censors who would make a recommendation to the membership. Members present at a regular meeting then voted on the new member. From 1904 to 1919, only one proposed individual was not accepted into membership because she was not registered in the state.

Counted among their members was Miss Linda Richards, America's first trained nurse, who was residing in the community in 1907. She was the Superintendent of Nurses at the Michigan Asylum and established a school of nursing at the institution. It was to Linda Richards that we owe the system of charting and maintaining individual medical records and the wearing of uniforms.

Dues were $1 initially. When the constitution and bylaws were revised in 1918, dues were increased to $2 with the understanding that the *American Journal of Nursing* would be included in the annual fee. By the close of 1917, membership had grown to 59 despite the fact that three members left to serve with the Red Cross during World War I and "five have left the field of nursing to enlist on the sea of matrimony" (GNAK Annual Report, January 30, 1918).

Registry and Salaries

The most immediate concern of the GNAK was to establish a directory/registry. A committee approached Dr. Della Pierce, one of the early female physicians in Kalamazoo and sister to the GNAK president, to maintain a directory. She graciously accepted and performed this function for many years. The GNAK set the salaries that nurses from the directory could charge. In 1904, $18.00 was charged for a week of providing standard care with $21.00 for contagious cases. At this time, most nursing was in the form of private duty. In 1907, nurses were supplied for 245 cases (143 in Kalamazoo and 102 out of town). By 1918, salaries were increased to $30.00 for regular and obstetric cases and $35.00 for contagion (GNAK minutes, June 26, 1918).

Activities

The major activities of GNAK centered on promoting fellowship among nurses. Meetings generally focused on business followed by a program and refreshments. Program topics varied widely, but included readings and discussion of published articles and talks on nursing or health care topics delivered by experts. Also included were discussions of registration, suffrage, the workings of the Red Cross, the activities of the MSNA and the ANA, and a tribute to Florence Nightingale on the occasion of that lady's death.

In 1911, GNAK proposed to fund a bed for sick nurses at Bronson Hospital. Funds remaining in the treasury after expenses were used for this purpose with special assessments from time to time. Over the years other special contributions were made to address child welfare, provide a "Thanksgiving offering" to the county visiting nurse, support the Red Cross, and send packages to France during WWI.

The GNAK was also concerned about the image of nurses. When an article in the *Gazette Telegraph* headed "Kalamazoo nurse advocates free love" appeared, the GNAK members were quick to respond that the writer was not a member, not known to the registrar, nor acquainted with any graduate or practical nurse of this city (GNAK minutes, August 30, 1916).

Joining MSNA

GNAK first hosted the MSNA convention in 1916. Although individual members of GNAK joined the MSNA and attended the annual meetings, specific steps were not taken until 1917 to become a district of MSNA. A circular entitled 'How Can Michigan Nurses Help with the War Relief' that urged nurses to join the state association (GNAK minutes, Sept. 26, 1917) provided the incentive to explore membership. When a new constitution and bylaws were written, Berrien, Van Buren, Cass, and St. Joseph counties were included. In May of 1918, the GNAK became the 5th District of the Michigan State Nurses Association.

Based on the minutes of the Graduate Nurses Association of Kalamazoo, minutes 1904-1918.

1914-1923

by Tom Bissonnette

The Great War, Public Health Nursing Begins, Women Win the Right to Vote

America's relationships with other countries were attracting considerable attention during this decade. In Europe, World War I, also known as the Great War, started in 1914, and in Mexico, the Mexican Revolution occurred. Americans initially did not want to get involved in World War I, although America did support the Allies in their fight against Germany, Austria, Hungary, Bulgaria, and Turkey. The United States finally entered the war in 1917, and it ended in 1918, with the Treaty of Versailles being signed in 1919. The Allied Powers of the United States, Great Britain, Japan, Italy, Russia, France, Belgium, Serbia, and Montenegro were victorious. And on April 28, 1919, the Michigan State Nurses Association held a memorial service for the fifteen Michigan nurses who had made the supreme sacrifice in the service of their country.

Domestic matters were also of grave concern during this decade. The public's health had been threatened for decades by tuberculosis and concerted, organized treatment and prevention efforts were being led by the American Red Cross and a few state anti-tuberculosis societies. And then the Great Flu Pandemic of 1918 hit, and between 30 to 50 million people died worldwide. Americans buried 200,000 flu victims just in October of 1918!

Influenza had a tremendous effect on Americans both at home and in Europe, as World War I was a potent carrier. As soldiers returned home and others left for the front, they carried the virus with them. Entire ships were infected. It is estimated that half of the American soldiers in Europe were killed by the flu.

Many Michigan nurses provided nursing service during World War I, and many returned to civilian life and joined the American Legion, and later, the National Organization of World War Nurses, in order to preserve some of their war time associations. Nurses were the only women eligible to be members of the American Legion at that time. A poem passed along by

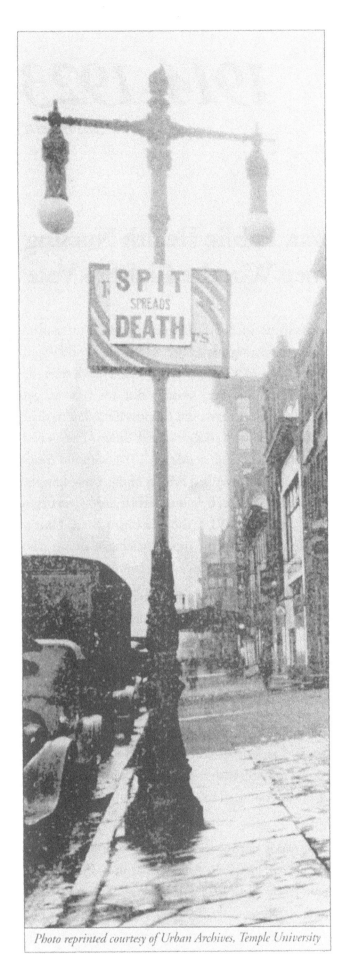

Michigan nurses which reflects the hard times and the humor of soldiers who endured the war and the flu follows:

Before I fell a victim

To the wiles of Spanish flu

I'd gathered from the posters

And from certain movies, too,

That when it came to nurses

You always woke to view

Some peach from Ziegfeld's Follies

Who slipped the pills to you.

I've read the artful fiction

About the angels fair

Who sat beside your pillow

And stroked your fevered hair

And made you kind of careless

How long you lingered there

In the radiant effulgence

Of a lovely baby stare.

That may be so in cases,

The way it is in plays

But mine was no white lady

Of lilting roundelays;

For while I was a blessé

The nurse who met my gaze

Was Private Pete Koszolski

Who hadn't shaved for days.

So wrote Lieutenant John Pierre Roche, 87th Division, US Army, during the dark days of 1917. Hundreds and thousands of American soldiers, sailors, and marines who served during World War I were more fortunate. They "woke to view" not a "peach from Ziegfeld's Follies" but what was a much more welcome sight, a graduate nurse, serene and efficient. Of course, had Lt. Roche known it, even the hands of Private Koszolski had been trained by one of those same nurses.

More people died in a single year from the flu than in four years of the bubonic plague (1347-1351). At the peak of the flu pandemic, one-fifth of the world's population was infected. Some of the stories during this pandemic are frightening. Four women were playing bridge late into the evening one night; three of them were dead by the next morning. Schools, lodges, and bowling alleys were closed. Churches opened for fifteen minute funerals until there were so few undertakers and grave diggers that bodies were stacked in storage until enough men were well enough to bury them. Contact with other people was avoided unless absolutely necessary.

The flu was very selective, killing healthy adults and leaving alone the old, infirm, and very young. In one report, a house was found full of dead adults with a young child, alive, sitting in the middle of the bodies.

A popular jump rope rhyme during this era was:

I had a little bird,

Its name was Enza,

I opened the window,

And in-flu-enza.

There was no time to diagnose flu symptoms as people often died within hours of being infected. The most common cause of death from the flu before this pandemic was pneumonia. This virus never allowed a victim to live long enough to develop classic pneumonia, as those infected died from uncontrolled hemorrhaging that rapidly filled their lungs.

And even through the flu pandemic and World War I, women won the right to vote in 1920.

Young people had quickly grown tired of the war and when the war had ended, and the flu had subsided, looked for some means of enjoying themselves. Many whites became interested in African American culture.

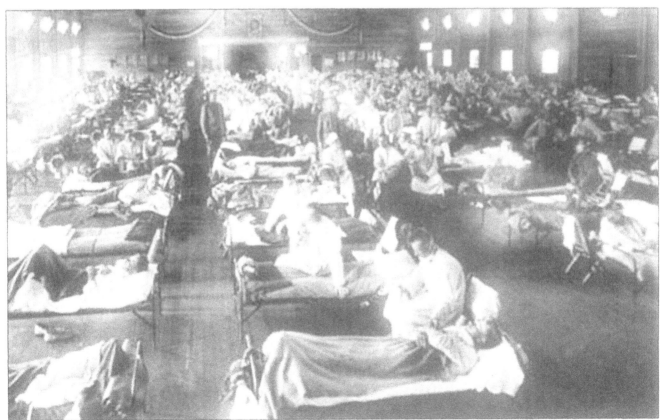

Photo courtesy of Otis Historical Archives of the National Museum of Health & Medicine

The flu panemic of 1918 began in the trenches of World War 1 and quickly spread worldwide. Between 30-50 million people died worldwide.

Harlem nightclubs thrived and spotlighted numerous artists such as jazz musicians Louis Armstrong and Duke Ellington. The "roaring twenties" had begun.

Michigan nurses began this decade by forming the State League of Nursing Education, forerunner of the Michigan League for Nursing, at the 1913 Michigan State Nurses Association annual meeting. Marie Belle McCabe, an instructor at the Grand Rapids Junior College, describes why the State League of Nursing Education was formed in her 1930 history of **Nursing in Michigan**: "The League was organized for the sole purpose of studying nursing fields with the object of planning a proficient education for any demands. It is to the glory of the nurses of Michigan that they have never been satisfied with the condition they found. The attitude has always been one of improvement. 'Better standards of nursing' was, and is, the constant battle cry."

During the Michigan State Nurses Association annual meeting in 1914, member dues were increased to $2.00. Districts were formalized and numbered in 1915 to create order and to give recognition to the groups of nurses who were geographically organized prior to the creation of the MSNA, as well as to those groups who were gathering in an organized way following the creation of the state association. Detroit District, which organized on November 13, 1902, was given the honor of being numbered as District 1 of the MSNA. Grand Rapids and Bay City (1904), with Jackson (1906), Saginaw (1908), Houghton (1913), and Lansing (1914) all formed distinct entities prior to the Association's numbering of districts in 1915.

Once MSNA began to number and recognize geographically distinct districts, several formed in the second decade of the Association: Flint (1916), Port Huron (1917), Battle Creek and Kalamazoo (1918), Muskegon, Ann Arbor, and Marquette (1919), and Traverse City (1923). Districts were assessed MSNA dues of $1.50 for each district member in 1923.

Membership for our youthful association was a concern, as well as support for women's issues of the time. MSNA became an associate member of the Michigan

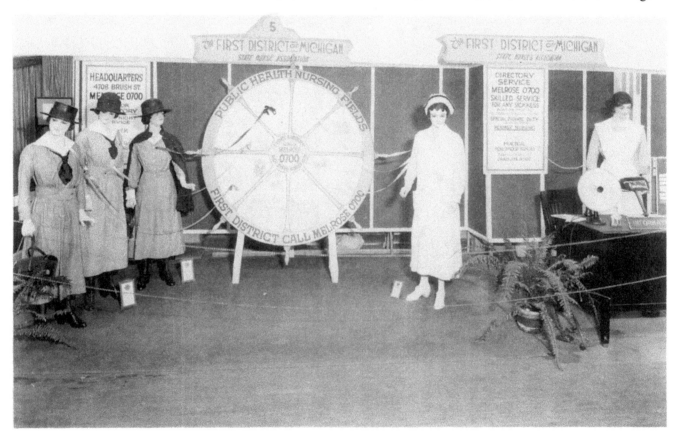

Detroit District, which organized on November 13, 1902, was given the honor of being numbered as District 1 of the MSNA.

Business and Professional Women's Association in 1920, and in the same year affiliated with the League of Women Voters. Nurses were solicited to contribute a day's salary to the Nurses Relief Fund in 1921. A membership drive was begun in 1922 with the goal of 3,000 nurse members by the end of the year. It is not known if the membership drive achieved its goal.

Legislative activity continued for the young Association, as an attempt was made to amend the registration statute in June of 1919. There was a nursing shortage as a result of the flu epidemic, and legislators sought to solve it with a "Junior Nurse Bill." With very short notice, a group of thirty nurses and several interested friends gathered in Lansing for a public hearing before the legislature to protest against this bill. The bill was withdrawn when the sponsors of the bill were assured by the Association that, after a proper study of the situation, a very definite provision would be made to increase the ranks of nurses or their attendants. A special committee was formed to address this matter.

After careful study, the committee found that the New York "Trained Attendant Act" was the most acceptable plan for Michigan. In 1921, the Nurses Registration Act was amended to include the registration of trained attendants.

According to the 1921 amendment, a trained attendant was a person who had taken a course in a hospital which provided definite training to this end. The curriculum was defined by the State Board of Registration and applicants were required to pass an examination before the State Board.

In 1923 an attempt was made to pass what was known as the "Epsie Bill," (House Bill 477) which proposed the following changes:

1. Substituted for the words "Trained Attendant" those of "Junior Nurses."

2. Eliminated the clause requiring the annual renewal of nurse registration.

3. Took away the authority of the Board of Registration to accredit schools of nursing.

4. Abolished the office of the inspector of the schools of nursing.

Through the efforts of the Association's legislative committee, a public hearing was held, and this bill was killed in committee.

MSNA was very active in public health nursing, and became a corporate member of the National Organization for Public Health Nursing in 1916. A committee was also formed to establish a plan to submit a course in public health nursing at the University of Michigan, in 1917.

From the turn of the century, public health nursing was provided through collaboration between the American Red Cross and the Michigan Anti-Tuberculosis Societies, which had developed community nursing programs for the treatment of tuberculosis and other disorders. Registered nurses were paid from county funds and were under the supervision of the Michigan Department of Health. In 1927, a new bill was passed which allowed any township in Michigan to set aside monies to pay a nurse(s) strictly for public nursing.

It was the creation of a new division in the Department of Health, however, that laid the foundation for systemized public health nursing throughout Michigan. Beginning in 1921, the Bureau of Child Hygiene and Public Health Nursing had a widespread influence as nurses were put into counties where no nurses were available, health centers were established and baby classes held. The Bureau was also given the charge to prevent sickness and restrict the spread of contagious diseases.

Although tuberculosis had been a serious problem since the late 1800s, efforts to control the disease with statewide programs did not take place until 1908, when a state committee called the Michigan Association for the Prevention and Relief of Tuberculosis was formed. Our young registered nurses association, the Michigan State Nurses Association, was very interested in the Tuberculosis Association's first project, which was to arrange exhibits for the

Caring for the Community

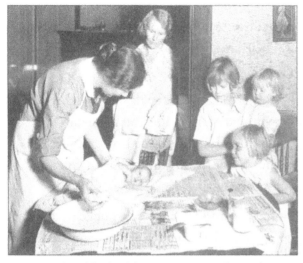 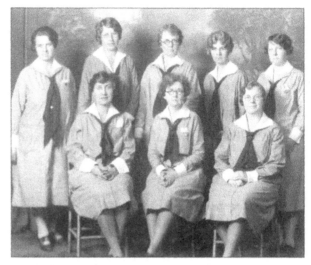

Systemized public health nursing in Michigan began in 1921 with the opening of the Bureau of Child Hygiene and Public Health Nursing. In succeeding years, the work of public health nurses resulted in increased child health, lower infant mortality, an increase in mothers surviving the birth of their babies, and a decrease in deaths from tuberculosis.

(Above l, ca. 1938) A visiting nurse instructs a family in neonatal care. (R, 1928) Nursing staff of the Department of Health and Safety, Saginaw. (Back l-r) School Nurses Augusta Ruede, Elsie Braun, Josephine Earley, Edith Vincent, and Edwina Nelson. (Front l-r) Prenatal Nurse Helen Albano, Supervisor of Nurses Mary McGovern, and Contagion Nurse Hettie Balhoff.

International Congress on Tuberculosis. The RNs donated money for the project and submitted a group picture and a resolution offering the support and cooperation of the nurses in any initiatives to control the disease.

The combination of nursing service, visiting nurses in the homes and the free clinics began to make a significant difference in Michigan. The Grand Rapids Anti-Tuberculosis Society saw deaths decrease from 307 in the three years before the Society was formed to 73 in the three years after the Society began. Their visiting nurse – their *one* visiting nurse – averaged 100 to 200 visits to tuberculosis patients per month with 73 cases under observation. The Detroit Society for the Study and Prevention of Tuberculosis employed four visiting nurses who taught and cared for all of the tuberculosis-stricken poor, free of charge.

Nurses offered a broad range of services. Patients in the early 1900s were not only given health instruction and care, but were also given milk tickets (by the quart) and eggs (by the dozen). And the nurses evaluated their tuberculosis teaching by four expert categories: careful cases, fairly careful cases, careless cases, and grossly careless.

By 1921, the Bureau of Child Hygiene and Public Health Nursing was deeply involved in four areas of community health:

1. Prenatal care

2. Infants from birth to two years of age

3. Children from two years to six years

4. Inspecting school children

Nurses visited 53 counties in 1921, teaching and explaining the need for good health within the communities. Schools of nursing were also contacted, so that new nurses were aware of the field of public health nursing. By 1922, the nurses had examined 736 under school age children, finding that 25.8 percent of them were underweight.

In 1929, over 500 nurses were employed in public health nursing. Children were healthier, the infant mortality rate had dropped, and more mothers survived the birth of their children. Though education classes were rejected at first by many communities, the nurses persevered and eventually won, as more and more patients began coming.

The victory did not come without cost. Many of the first visiting nurses contracted tuberculosis themselves and died. It was hazardous, exhausting work. Many of the nurses started out with a horse and buggy to travel to their patients. Yet the interest in public health nursing never waned among the nurses. Their work was making a significant difference in the lives of thousands of patients.

The nurse leaders of the young MSNA contributed mightily to the efforts of maintaining and improving the health of the Michigan public, as evidenced in the article below.

The School Nurse in Flint

By Ann Kettering Sincox

Flint, Michigan, is an industrial center which has had an exceedingly rapid growth. In 1900 it boasted of a population of 13,000; today the population is estimated at about 142,000.

The growth of the school population, of course, has been equally astounding. In 1914 there were 5,800 children in school, including the high school; today there are about 21,000.

The Flint Board of Education has conducted its own health work since 1913, with the appointment at that time of one school nurse. A medical director and a dentist were appointed in 1923. "The ultimate aim" as given by Dr. Eugene Pierce, Medical Director, and Miss Flora Burgdorf, RN, Supervisor of Nurses,

in an article entitled "Public School Health Departments in an Industrial Center," which appeared in the *Nation's Health* in 1927, was to see that the child was placed in the best school environment to secure the highest possible physical and mental development.

Eleven fresh air rooms were wholly maintained by the Board of Education, each with an enrollment of thirty pupils. The poorly nourished child, the tuberculosis contact, cardiac cases, and children recovering from recent operations or illness were admitted to these rooms. The cost of health work per pupil in 1926 was $1.41.

(Source: *The Michigan Nurse*, September 1928)

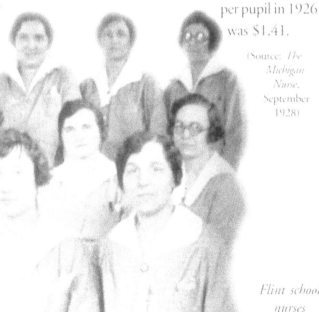

Flint school nurses

17

Lulu L. Cudney, RN

by Lisa Gottlieb-Kinnaird

Lulu L. Cudney's belief in service was reflected in her chosen profession as a registered nurse. A charter member of the Michigan State Nurses Association, Cudney was born to pioneer parents in Nebraska in 1874.

A graduate of Butterworth Hospital School of Nursing's (Grand Rapids) 1898 class, she remained active in her profession for almost 68 years, continuing to take cases when she was 88 years old.

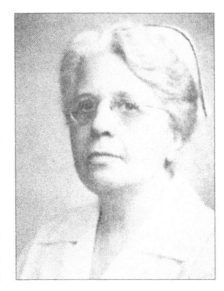

I have loved my profession as God's work for humanity.

-Lulu L. Cudney

Nurses today who are debating whether they should join their professional association can learn from Cudney's positive spin on the benefits of membership. Said she, "I would rather have gone without a new dress than to miss a year of membership."

Cudney's nursing career encompassed years when significant health care advances changed the face of nursing and lengthened life spans. These included diphtheria vaccinations, the use of silver nitrate in the eyes of newborn babies to prevent disease, and the introduction of intensive care units for post-operative patients.

She served as a nurse during World War I and survived the flu pandemic of 1918, where she saw 125 patients die of the deadly disease in one day.

As the years slipped by, she witnessed a change in the role of the registered nurse from bedside to hospital nursing.

Nonetheless, she continued to recognize the value of the registered nurse, no matter what the setting. Cudney felt that when the public went to visit a sick relative or family member in the hospital, "they expect to see registered nurses" at the bedside caring for their loved one.

In 1956, Cudney worked closely with Darling Freight, Inc. of Grand Rapids to establish a nursing scholarship program for students within the nine states in which the company operated.

Under the terms of the program, four nursing scholarships were awarded each year to selected schools of nursing within the nine-state area. Each scholarship was for three years' duration – the length of time necessary to complete a diploma program in nursing.

Cudney was no stranger to the problem of nursing tasks being performed by those less qualified and the struggles of nurses for recognition and greater control of their profession. In an era of registered nurses and licensed practical nurses, Cudney feared that the licensed practical nurse would become the "important one in the hospital if the registered nurses do not take leadership."

Surely Lulu L. Cudney would look on the efforts of today's nurses for increased education and autonomy with approval.

Excerpted from *The Michigan Nurse*, May-June 1961 and a 1952 newspaper article.

Lulu L. Cudney
Remembers

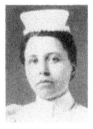

Lulu L. Cudney, RN

Early nursing with the training of nurses was established primarily for the care of the sick, which was bedside nursing…In 1890 and later the training period was two years…Students in senior years were expected to serve in the capacity of a special private nurse…It was quite common for students to be sent out to homes with doctors on obstetrical and surgical cases…We also had our share of contagious and medical cases in homes…Those were the horse and buggy days with long rides into the country to patients…No ambulances, no comfortable transportation; we went as best we could, equipped to meet the emergency in lamp lighted rooms.

Our hours were long and confining…I recall being sent in 1898 to help our one visiting nurse, and that was 12-hour duty for a limited time…We had two hours off duty, and slept as we could at night.

Student nurses were paid a small sum of money …The class of 1898 received $6 per month and were required to make and furnish their own uniforms…The second year we were to receive $8 per month, but the hospital started furnishing the uniforms, and there was some discussion about discontinuing the $8 per month…We accepted the change, however, with no petition being circulated for signing, as might be done in these present days.

As time passed more graduates were employed in the hospitals…School nursing was established in the early 1900s…Visiting nurses for city needs were increased…Dietitians became a part of the hospital staff to replace students who had formerly been in charge of food service.

Bells were answered by nurses and also by those serving their probationary time of three months …It was not unusual for the superintendent of nurses making her morning calls, upon seeing a call light, to step into the room to ask what was wanted.

We were a family in those good old days… However, I would not wish for the nursing profession to return to the past…I love to think of the firm foundation laid by the pioneers in the nursing profession, even before there was any organization in existence.

I was proud to be a charter member of the state association and to become an RN in Michigan …My registry number is 829, and I am still using it as a private duty nurse, for which I am humbly grateful.

(Source: *The Michigan Nurse*, January 1954)

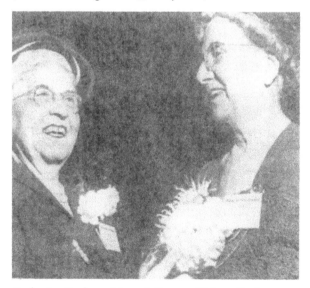

Lulu L. Cudney (r) and Emma Nelson Embry were honored during MSNA's 50th Anniversary Convention as the oldest active nurses in Michigan.

1924-1933

by Tom Bissonnette

Timeline

Nursing Education Improves, the Great Depression Creates Unemployment

The roaring twenties were in full roar at the start of this decade, with flapper dresses being tremendously popular by 1925. Americans were enjoying the "good life" following the horrors of the previous ten years. One could now dial telephone numbers unassisted by using a rotary dial phone. Secretary of State Bainbridge Colby certified the 19th Amendment to the US Constitution which gave women the right to vote in 1920. Canadian biochemists Frederick Banting and Charles Best discovered insulin on July 27, 1921. This discovery was followed by Alexander Fleming's identification of a bacteria killing compound in London on September 15, 1928 – penicillin. Sigmund Freud presented the Ego and the Id in 1923.

American manufacturing was at full throttle in the '20s: US Steel offered an eight hour work day in 1923, and Ford offered the Model A in 1927, receiving over 50,000 orders. Yet by 1930, the average American annual salary was $1,368, and in 1932 one out of every four American families was on governmental relief aid. This occurred because of the stock market crash on October 29, 1929, commonly known as "Black Tuesday," when the Great Depression began. Unemployment skyrocketed – a quarter of the workforce was without jobs by 1933, and many Americans were homeless. President Herbert Hoover attempted to manage the crisis but was unable to improve the situation. In 1932, Franklin Delano Roosevelt was elected president, and he promised a "New Deal" for the American people. Congress created the Works Progress Administration which offered work relief for thousands.

And nurses, who were in such demand just a few years earlier, found themselves unemployed.

At the start of this third decade for the Michigan State Nurses Association, all attention was upon improving nursing education. Shirley Titus, the second

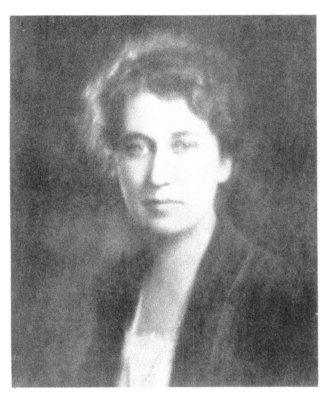

In 1928, MSNA Second Vice President Shirley Titus spoke out on the need for more and better trained nurses.

vice president of the Association who was also the president of the Michigan League of Nursing Education, led the charge. Ms. Titus, who was Director of the School of the Nursing as well as University Hospital in Ann Arbor, described "Salient Problems of Contemporary Nursing Education" in the February 1928 issue of *The Michigan Nurse*. She makes recommendations for the improvement of nursing education in a speech to the Michigan Federation of Women's Clubs that nurse educators will find current today:

"I say, therefore, we need many more nurses, a distinctly better type of nurse, and infinitely better prepared nurses. How then shall we secure them?

First, through a clear recognition that the present form, or system, of nurse education is in a large measure inadequate and obsolete and needs a thorough renovation from attic to cellar.

Second, that the greatest role of the nurse today is that of a health educator rather than a remedial agent.

Third, the preparation of the nurse for her life's work is an educational process, rather than a mere training in handicraft, and constitutes part and parcel of the general field of education, which fact clearly implies that educators must of necessity turn their attentions to nursing education as well as to any other form of educational problem.

Fourth, nursing schools should receive state aid in the way of financial support, and private endowments for schools of nursing should be encouraged.

Fifth, there should be a distinct movement toward modifying or abolishing the apprenticeship system on which nursing now rests; the state or private endowment should pay part of the bill for educating nurses and the student nurse herself should pay for her share of this expense in dollars and cents instead of through service rendered to the hospital.

Sixth – and perhaps most important of all – every means must be used to interest the public in the problem of nursing education in order that the foregoing goals may be reached in the shortest possible time."

At the time Ms. Titus was writing, there were about 2,000 accredited nurse training schools in the United States, and about 2,000 unaccredited schools. This compares to the total of *fifteen* schools in 1885! Hospitals had discovered the tremendous economic value of having their own "training schools for nurses," and practically every hospital had their own school. Nursing students were offered "training" free of charge in exchange for mopping, scrubbing, and polishing floors during 12-14 hour work days with ever-thinning "instruction." Nursing students were not paid for this work.

As Shirley Titus remarked, "You wonder…why women of intelligence and refinement went into nursing under such conditions, why they were willing to pay such a heavy price for becoming nurses." The only vocations open to women had been only four in number: marriage, old-maidism, teaching, and nursing. During this time, the vast majority of nursing schools admitted students who had only one or two years of high school education. Within every one hundred hours of training, students received seven hours of theory and ninety-three hours of practicum!

During this clarion call for nursing education reform, the Great Depression struck. Janet M. Geister, Headquarters Director of the American Nurses Association, is quoted in the December 1930 issue of *The Michigan Nurse*:

"Unemployment is our greatest problem at present time. We are acutely aware of it and are giving it our major attention. The reasons for unemployment furnish us with a basis for attacking the problem, but it is something that will require the attention and effort of every individual nurse, as well as organized nursing, if any headway is to be made in its solution.

Nursing is at a crossroads. We are faced with too many nurses within the profession and we are graduating too many nurses each year. There has been poor distribution of nursing service, and the fluctuation in the stock market has made the situation more acute. A change in the types of nursing service offered to the public is essential if any improvement in unemployment is to be expected. The use of graduate nurse service in the hospital to replace that of student nurse service has been suggested. The study of the use of the graduate staff in the hospital is to be the next study and additional studies of hourly and group nursing are to be made also."

Olive Sewell, RN, the Michigan State Nurses Association's second Executive Secretary, comments on the Michigan experience of unemployed nurses in the same issue of *The Michigan Nurse*:

"It should be interesting and reassuring to private duty nurses throughout Michigan to know that not only the nation but the state as well is making every effort to lessen the existing unemployment. Several schools have decided to take only one new class this year (1930), substituting graduate nursing service for student nursing. This will not only reduce the output of nurses, but will give immediate employment to some of those who are now in the overcrowded private duty group."

The combination of the call for nursing education reform and the economy seems to have initiated the educational reform in our schools of nursing. A worsening nurse employment picture is evidenced in this short burst from Ms. Sewell in January 1931:

"Think twice before spending your money and energy in seeking a job away from your home community. Leaders are recommending that for the next months, at least, you stay in the locality where you are known by doctors, hospitals, registry, and patients. Do not go elsewhere in the expectation of finding something better to

Those Who Marched
Olive Sewell, RN

by Lisa Gottlieb-Kinnaird

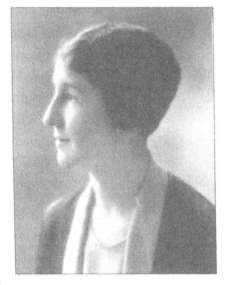

Olive Sewell was born in Minnesota and received her nursing education at the Minneapolis City Hospital School of Nursing, graduating in 1915. During World War I she served in Warsaw, Poland then spent seven years in Serbia working for the Child Welfare Commission. When peace was declared, she returned to the United States where she became head supervisor of Grace Hospital, Detroit then director of the nursing school at Sparrow Hospital, Lansing. She was appointed Executive Secretary of MSNA on January 1, 1930.

In a time when the nursing profession was struggling to reorganize and modernize its methods of education and service, Olive Sewell worked tirelessly to advance the association and educate the membership, allied professions and the public about the role of the nurse. Under her direction, MSNA headquarters moved from a corner desk to a business suite and assumed a powerful leadership in nursing and health affairs. Largely through her efforts, the Michigan State Public Health Organization was born.

With spirit and optimism, Olive Sewell fostered the trailblazing mentality which has become a hallmark of the Michigan Nurses Association. During her tenure, the 8-hour day for nurses became generally accepted, state sections for industrial, staff and office nurses were organized, and the number of district associations grew from seventeen to forty-four. She aided greatly in the formation of local councils for the Michigan Nursing Council for War Service.

A woman of culture and refinement, Olive Sewell loved books, music, art and travel. Single all her life, she nonetheless adopted a daughter, Mary.

Olive Sewell died unexpectedly on July 10, 1944. A wealth of condolence notes and reminiscenses from nursing leaders throughout the country indicate the high esteem in which they held Olive Sewell and her remarkable achievements on behalf of the nursing profession.

Excerpted from *The Michigan Nurse,* October, 1944.

do. Almost certainly you will meet in the next town conditions similar to your own, of a decrease in the number of calls for nurses over that of the past several years, and an increase in the short-duration call of from one to three days."

The change for the vast majority of nurses employed in the private duty sector to "hourly" nursing was now occurring in the profession as a result of the economy. An Association member, Winifred Rand, describes the change in a February 1932 article of *The Michigan Nurse*:

"It is apparent that in certain types of sickness a patient does not need skilled nursing care for eight, twelve, or twenty-four hours in the day but does need a nurse for one or two hours in the day. The patient wants a nurse for a short time …to do for her what a private duty nurse in some types of cases does for the whole day, and she may want this nurse at a specified time in the day."

As Ms. Rand elaborates in her article, many patients who needed nursing services for a small part of the day had paid for an entire day of nursing services as they didn't have any other option for obtaining nursing services. This resulted in a high price as well as frustration for both the patient and nurse. The nurse was often under utilized for nursing services and the patient was paying for unneeded nursing services. The economy drove nursing to present other options, and this included "hourly" or "appointment" nursing, paid at an hourly rate.

Growing the Association's membership remained a priority during this decade. In 1926, 869 (36%) of 2,414 members did not renew their Association membership. In 1927, 1,090 (31%) of 3,516 members did not renew. Given this nearly 1/3 non-renewal rate, the Association began a formal dues invoice system in 1929. Additionally, an analysis of non-Association members by Association district was done in 1930 and given to districts to extend invitations to these non-member nurses. The number of non-members by district included:

Ann Arbor	.230
Battle Creek	209
Lansing	95
Bay City	64
Marquette	70
Flint	267
Muskegon	65
Detroit	1,614
Port Huron	36
Grand Rapids	305
Saginaw	130
Grayling	9
St. Joseph	59
Houghton	68
Traverse City	53
Jackson	116

The number of nurses registered in Michigan in 1932 included 10,716 who re-registered, and an additional 1,140 newly registered for that year, for a total of 11,856. Membership in the Michigan State Nurses Association in 1932 had declined in every district since 1931, except for Ann Arbor, Detroit, Kalamazoo, and Muskegon. Along with the Association, the Michigan Board of Registration of Nurses had called for a decrease in the number of students admitted to nursing schools for the 1932 school year due to the economy and resulting massive unemployment of nurses. As such, the number of students admitted to Michigan nursing schools in 1931 was 1,109, and in 1932 the number was 285! Also of note, in 1930 the Board and the Association urged the voluntary raising of standards for entrance into schools of nursing to that of high school graduation. Of the 1,109 students admitted in 1931, all but eleven students had high school diplomas.

The Association remained involved in legislation during this decade. As M. Eleanor McGarvah, a registered nurse and attorney, wrote in the annual meeting edition of *The Michigan Nurse* in 1931:

"In 1927 the legislative committee submitted a new Registration Bill known as Senate Bill No. 270 to the legislature. This bill was a vast improvement on the 1921 statute (Trained

Detroit Hourly Nursing Service

What?

Graduate Nursing Service in the home by the hour instead of by the day for patients of wealth and moderate means alike, who do not need continuous nursing.

Why?

1. Hourly nursing permits a better distribution of professional nursing service.

2. Present day living demands this changing order.

3. Hourly nursing helps to answer the question "How can the high cost of sickness be met?"

Where can it be obtained?

This service is offered jointly by the Detroit District Nurses Association and the Visiting Nurse Association of Detroit.

$2.00 for the first hour and 50 cents for each additional ½ hour or fraction thereof.

51 Warren Avenue West

GLENDALE 1600. After 8:00 P. M., also Sundays and Holidays—GLENDALE 1981-2081.

*Hourly Nursing is the Response to a Long
Felt Need of the Physician*

Attendant Act). Every effort had been made by the Association to advise all persons who would be interested in its contents, and apparently all were in favor and had promised to support the bill. A request had been made in this bill for a board of ten members, seven of which were nurses, two physicians, and one educator. At the last minute, the legislative committee was advised that their bill could not be passed unless there was a change made to the character of the board. As an alternative the nurses were offered a board consisting of three physicians and two nurses. Rather than accept this offer, the committee requested that their bill be suppressed."

Additional legislative activity to improve Michigan's Nurse Registration Act continued in 1930 and 1931, with an inability to reach consensus with the Michigan Medical Association and the Michigan Hospital Association resulting in the lack of any successful legislation.

Those Who Marched

Mary Staines Foy, RN

by Lisa Gottlieb-Kinnaird

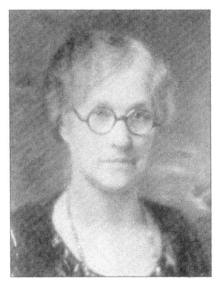

Known as the "Dean of Battle Creek Nurses," Mary Staines Foy was a pioneer whose nursing career spanned 70 years. Born April 21, 1863 in Bushnell, Michigan, she attended the Greenville Public Schools and Battle Creek College. In 1878, she was hired by the Battle Creek Sanitarium to perform nursing duties.

The Sanitarium organized a School of Nursing in 1884, and Mary Staines Foy enrolled in the first class. However, due to her responsibilities as office assistant to Dr. John Harvey Kellogg, the facility's medical director, she was unable to graduate until 1890.

Following her graduation she supervised various medical departments in the facility and subsequently became principal of the School of Nursing, Director of Nursing, and dean and director of the School of Nursing of Battle Creek College, associated with the Battle Creek Sanitarium and Hospital. The *Sanitarium News* reported, "There was the greatest need for workers with ability, initiative, resourcefulness, dependability, and above all good judgment and a large fund of common sense, and in these essential qualities, Mary Staines Foy filled the bill to an unusual degree." More than 2,000 nursing students owe their training to this remarkable woman.

Recognizing the strength of nurses working together to advance their profession, Mary Staines Foy was active in many nursing organizations. She became an ANA member in 1900 and was a charter member of the Michigan Nurses Association and a member of the International Council of Nursing since its organization. She attended the first mass meeting of American nurses in Chicago in 1893 when the American Society of Superintendents of Training Schools for Nurses (later the National League of Nursing Education) was formed. She joined the Michigan League of Nursing Education in 1913. She belonged to the Michigan Board of Registration of Nurses and served as vice president and secretary in that organization.

She was awarded an honorary degree of Master of Liberal Arts from Olivet College in 1925 in recognition of her contribution to human welfare.

Active in retirement into her 85th year, she served the Sanitarium Nurses Alumnae Association as their corresponding secretary and wrote their quarterly newsletter.

Excerpted from *The Michigan Nurse*, April 1928, September 1933, and May 1948.

1934-1943

by Jess Merrill

Timeline

National Labor Relations Act Created, Red Cross Seeks Nurses for War Effort

The Great Depression had a firm grip on America in 1934, easing in 1938 when the industrialized world began to prepare for the upcoming war in Europe.

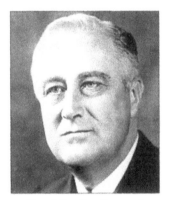

Franklin D. Roosevelt

The Social Security Act was signed into law in 1935, and the first checks were distributed in 1937. According to President Franklin D. Roosevelt, the cornerstone of the New Deal was the Social Security Act. Social Security established a system that provided old-age pensions for workers, survivor's benefits for victims of industrial accidents, unemployment insurance, and aid for dependant mothers and children, the blind and physically disabled. The program was funded in large part by taxes on the earnings of current workers, with a single fixed rate for all regardless of income. To President Roosevelt, these limitations on the programs were compromises to ensure passage.

The New Deal included a large number of programs designed to promote economic recovery and increase domestic employment. Among these was the Civilian Conservation Corps (CCC). This environmental program put 2.5 million unmarried men to work maintaining and restoring forests, beaches and parks. They earned $1 a day but received free board and job training. From 1934 to 1937 this program funded similar programs for 8,500 women. The CCC taught men and women how to live independently and provided job skills to take them into the mainstream workforce. By 1936, America's economic recovery was well underway with unemployment at 17 percent.

It was during the New Deal that organized labor made greater gains than at any previous time in American history. The National Labor Relations Act

(NLRA), also known as the Wagner Act, enacted in 1935, defined unfair labor practices, gave workers the right to bargain through unions of their own choice and prohibited employers from interfering with union activities. It also created the National Labor Relations Board to supervise collective bargaining, administer elections and ensure workers the right to choose the organization that should represent them.

The concepts of unionism and collective bargaining were points of heated contention among Michigan nurses. In the June, 1935 issue of *The Michigan Nurse*, editor Olive Sewell, RN, writes,

> "…It is inconceivable that, in any situation where the welfare of patients and the interests of the sick are at stake, professional nurses should seriously consider forming, or participating in, organizations which accept as a principle 'a collective withdrawal from work' even as a 'last resort.' An arbitrary limitation of hours controlled by law violates the whole spirit of nursing, as the comfort of the patient is the nurse's first consideration. However, an attempt should be made to approach reasonable working conditions by encouraging, where possible, in the interest of the patient as well as the nurse, an eight-hour day for those employed on a daily basis, and a forty-eight hour week for those employed on a weekly or monthly schedule."

General Motors recognized the United Auto Workers Union in February 1937, following strikes at assembly plants in Flint. Not quite three months later, in an incident to become known as "The Battle of the Overpass," Walter Reuther and a group of UAW supporters, fresh from having organized GM and Chrysler, attempted to distribute leaflets at the Ford Motor Company's River Rouge plant and were beaten by Ford Service Department guards.

Because of incidents such as these, unionism had developed a reputation that was synonymous with hostility and violence. In the following years that reputation as well as the concept of a strike and ensuing

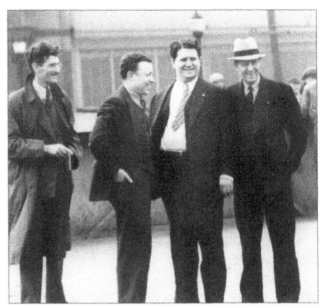

Photo courtesy of Walter P. Reuther Library, Wayne State University

An attempt was made to organize workers at the Ford Motor Company River Rouge Plant by (l-r) Robert Kanter, Walter Reuther, Richard Frankensteen, and J.J. Kennedy. Although organized labor began to make great strides during this decade, organizing RNs was considered to violate the spirit of nursing.

"patient abandonment," would play a part in nurses' objections to participation in collective bargaining activities.

The Wages and Hours (later Fair Labor Standards) Act was passed in June of 1938, banning child labor and setting the 40-hour work week. The Act went into effect in October 1940, and was upheld by the Supreme Court in February of 1941. MSNA appointed a committee in 1939 to secure information for the betterment of conditions of employment for hospital staff nurses. Henry Ford finally recognized the UAW in June of 1941.

Mrs. James K. Watkins, Chairman, Sustaining Members, wrote in her column SOPHN NEWS (State Organization of Public Health Nurses), in March 1936.

> "Individuals working alone progress slowly, but individuals banded together can work miracles … The greatest development of modern nursing has undoubtedly been in the field of Public Health. Public Health Nursing is an organized

community service rendered by especially prepared graduate nurses to the individual, the family, the community. Therefore, it is definitely a service to the layman and therefore he should be the one most interested in its promotion. The prime requirement is that 'the people' of a county or group of counties see their need and earnestly desire help in their health problems. Never before in Michigan have laymen had so great an opportunity to help themselves to health as now. There is as yet a chasm between what is known concerning health and what is being preached – this demands a program of education which the informed layman is peculiarly able to present to his community. An entire day is being given to the subject of lay participation in this Statewide Health Program, at the Annual Convention of the three State Nursing Organizations, to be held at Traverse City, May 21, 22, 23, 1936. This is your opportunity to acquaint yourself with this field of possible lay endeavor. A sample of questions to be considered in a round table discussion by the Committee includes:

- How can an advisory lay committee help to obtain an adequate community nursing program?

- How can we discover the outstanding health problems in our community?

- What can the layman do to reduce the tuberculosis and communicable disease rate?

- How will the Social Security Act benefit our community health program?

You are most cordially urged to be present especially on Thursday, May 21. Come and bring others from your community."

The concept of lay participation in nursing as introduced in 1936 became well-embedded in the association. A lay advisory council was suggested for each district so the public could better understand nursing's agenda.

Miss Claribel Wheeler wrote for *The Michigan Nurse* a January 1941 article titled "Lay Participation in Nursing Education."

"…Leadership within the profession is, of course, essential, but in addition there must be a sympathetic, understanding public which stands ready to assist and support the professional group. Education for any profession is a public responsibility, whether it is preparation for teaching, law, medicine, or nursing…The values of lay membership on a school committee are:

1. They interpret to the public the professional point of view as well as the needs of the school and the nursing service.

2. Their point of view cannot be challenged on the ground of self-interest or exaggerated professionalism, and [they] bring a fresh, unbiased point of view to the committee.

3. They give the program continuity in the community.

4. They see needs from the point of view of the consumer of nursing service.

One of the greatest needs that nursing has is that a large number of public spirited men and women may catch the vision of the changes that are necessary in nursing education, for only then will the future social order have its nursing needs more adequately cared for than they are today."

In a 1936 editorial in *The Michigan Nurse*, Norma Eskil, RN, chairman of the State Committee, Red Cross Nursing Service, wrote:

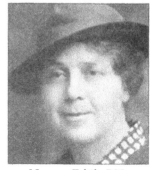

"Young Nurses! The Red Cross Calls You!

Nurses! Are you under forty, unmarried and in good health? If you have these requisites, why not

Norma Eskil, RN

Red Cross Seeks Nurses

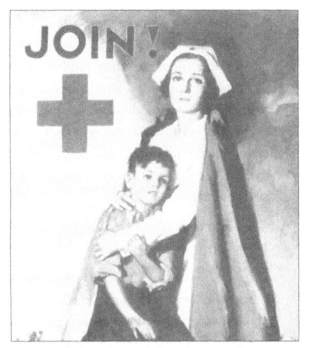

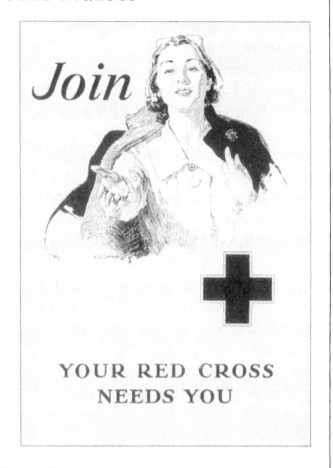

**YOUR RED CROSS
NEEDS YOU**

Concerned about the possibility of a national emergency, the American Red Cross sought to increase their enrollment. The Red Cross provided nursing services for the armed forces until the creation of the Army Nurse Cadet Corps.

enroll in the First Reserve of the Red Cross Nursing Service? Michigan's situation as far as the national Red Cross Nursing Service is concerned is as follows: On July 31, 1936, there were 552 nurses enrolled in the First Reserve. There should be at least 1,000 Michigan nurses enrolled. Surely there are that many who are eligible among our 6,000 members of the State Nurses Association."

Miss Bernadine Krause, RN, Hillsdale County Red Cross Committee member explained in *The Michigan Nurse*, January 1941:

"The Red Cross Nurse has always been a symbol of comfort in distress and aid in disaster. Throughout all the talk about National Defense, we have heard how the men are being prepared for the National Emergency [WWII]. People

are now asking about the nurses. Are they being prepared for the National Emergency, do we have enough and where are they?...The First Reserve with a present enrollment of nearly 17,000 nurses consists of unmarried registered nurses between the ages of 21 and 40.

...The Second Reserve consists of approximately 26,000 women who since enrolling have become ineligible for military duty. This group is a valuable reserve of qualified nurses whose skills and experience are immediately available to America's home defense.

...In case of war, the Red Cross has the responsibility of furnishing the necessary number of nurses to both the Army and Navy. At the present time, First Reserve nurses are being called so that approximately 4,000 will be in active service by July, 1941. These nurses will be placed in Army hospitals to look after the health of the thousands of new recruits coming in in the next few months. These nurses have the relative rank of Second Lieutenant in the Army."

It is important to note that the Red Cross was used as the supplier of nurses for the Armed Forces until the Army Nurse Cadet Corps was established. Also, nurses received only "relative" officer rank during WWII.

WWII had a revolutionary impact on nursing. A legislative milestone was reached when the US Congress appropriated a total of $4,750 million in 1941–1942 for nursing education under the Bolton bill. This is the first time the government recognized nurses as a group.

In 1944 President Roosevelt signed an executive order making nurses in the Army and Navy an integral part of the armed forces. After this, they received the same pay and privileges as other officers. During this period, practical nurses came into being and men started entering nursing in significant numbers (although not in the military). After the war, the GI Bill of Rights enabled many nurses who served their country to attend college and become better educated.

This was the dawn of new medicines like anti-histamines, cortisone and ACTH and radioactive isotopes. The war stimulated the production of penicillin, and, in 1943, the first penicillin injection was given using strict antiseptic technique. The yellow powder had to be reconstituted. The patient was given 5,000 units every two hours around the clock and showed remarkable improvement. It was hailed as a "wonder drug."

A brief review of MSNA district meetings in 1940 reveals a sense of civility, community service, and socializing among district members.

Battle Creek District

In July the Battle Creek District Nurses Association held a picnic at Forestina Monahan's Cottage, Fine Lake.

Fifty nurses were present September 9th at the Schuler Hotel in Marshall for a dinner and regular meeting. During the business meeting the nurses decided to make one hundred layettes as its part of the Calhoun County Red Cross War Relief quota.

Flint District

Feeling the need for closer cooperation and better understanding between the Department of Health, the Office nurses and Doctor's receptionists, the Department of Health invited them to attend a Dessert Luncheon. It was given in July at the new Women's Federation Club building. Sixty women, of whom about forty were graduate nurses, attended.

Houghton District

The Houghton District Nurses Association began the new season's activity with a business meeting followed by a tasty and beautifully served dinner at Keweenaw Golf Club.

The populace of Upper Michigan has been somewhat alarmed by the epidemic of poliomyelitis. Civic minded organizations banded together and within a surprisingly short time a respirator was purchased for St. Joseph's Hospital in Hancock.

Lenawee District

The first meeting of the Lenawee District Nurses Association was a banquet at "The Farm" near Onsted. About twenty were present. Mrs. Ann Pfister was toastmistress and presented the speaker, Mrs. Prentice, who gave a book review on **I Married an Adventurer.** A short business meeting followed.

Muskegon District

The program for the first fall meeting was limited to vacation or summer experiences of some of the nurses at home and abroad. Miss Mary Sagala spoke of her trip to New Orleans.

Mrs. Shaffer gave an account of her visit to Canada and the World's Fair.

These were typical District news reports in the October, 1940 issue of *The Michigan Nurse*. Districts used a social agenda to recruit and retain local members, and to encourage attendance at their meetings.

While the number of registered nurses in Michigan increased from approximately 13,000 in 1935 to approximately 20,000 in 1944 – nearly 54% – the MSNA membership rose disproportionately less, a little more than 18% to approximately 6,500 members.

By March 1947 there were 42 District Nurses Associations and 25 unaffiliated individual members in the Michigan State Nurses Association. Three districts; Delta, Dickinson, and Menominee had merged to form the Tri-County District. The Petoskey District had been discontinued, and Oceana had merged with Muskegon District.

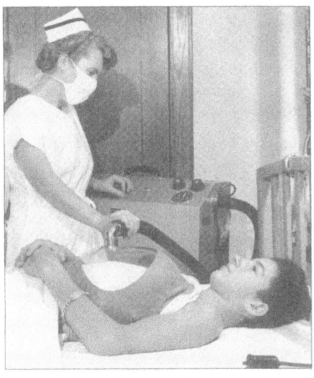

Low wages plus meals were typical remuneration for nurses in the '40s. Nursing was viewed as a service performed by dedicated individuals for whom the honor of belonging to the profession should be adequate recompense.

A perennial concern discussed within the Association was the service aspect of the nursing profession.

In October 1937, Edwina Wilkinson, assistant instructor, Harper School of Nursing, wrote in *The Stewardship of Nursing:*

"…A steward is one who waits on others, who manages for others, or, more important, one who holds something in trust…Demonstrating this concept of a nurse as a steward are the planks of the nursing platform, the same criteria which proclaim it a profession rather than an occupation or a trade. The purpose of nursing is primarily that of service; public interest is served before self interest, and the code of ethics practiced has been built up for the benefit of the patients. The aims lie in improving the health, safety, knowledge and goodness of the community. The degree of education, learning and skill must be sufficient to insure high-grade, efficient service. The watchword of nursing might well be 'obligation.' One's duty is not a daily eight hour fulfillment of an assignment, nor does nursing become drudgery, simply because its main intent is divorced from remuneration. At the recent Florence Nightingale memorial service, the Detroit group was admonished 'not to limit your giving to value for value expected in return.' Compensation then in this interpretation of nursing comes in the time expended, the talents which are employed and the opportunities which are used advantageously. If it is an emblem of service well rendered, then that compensation may well be the honor of belonging to the profession."

This attitude of nursing as selfless service without regard for financial compensation predates industrialized America, flies in the face of adequate compensation for highly educated professionals, and may well be the core of the general public's attitude that nursing, while emotionally highly valuable, may not have as great a value economically and should not necessarily be financially rewarding for the practitioner.

The public's attitude towards economic security for nurses is reflected in the following information:

"$4.00 per day plus two meals is the most common salary paid to graduate nurses employed in Detroit hospitals for temporary general staff duty on an eight hour service in 1940. Seven hospitals pay $4.00 plus two meals, four of them continuing this rate so long as the nurse is a temporary employee, whether for a long or short period. One hospital pays $4.50 per day and furnishes no meals, and one pays $5.00 per day."

The Michigan Nurse in October 1941, presented a Tentative Schedule of Salaries and Personnel Practices for Institutional Nurses and sent a letter to each member with an authorization letter enclosed. The authorization letter contained two propositions; proposition one asked members to approve and ratify the action of the Board of Directors establishing minimum salary standards and personnel policies. Proposition two asked for authorization for the Board of Directors of the Michigan State Nurses Association to act as the members' sole representative in negotiating salaries and minimum standards and personnel policies for the membership. The letter cited the National Labor Relations Act as the authority for setting up bargaining rights for the nursing profession and others.

Terms of this tentative schedule provided for a minimum recommended salary for a staff nurse at $160 per month without maintenance, and a $5.00 per month increase at the end of each year for a minimum of three years. Salary at the end of three years would be $175 per month without maintenance. Salary for an assistant head nurse was recommended at $170 per month, and $185 per month at the end of three years without maintenance. A head nurse could expect $180 per month and $195 per month after three years.

Nurses would not be required to take more than one meal a day in the hospital dining room, and the nurse would have the privilege of designating which meal she would take.

The hospital would at no time deduct from the nurse's pay check more than $10.00 per month provided the salary of the nursing staff remained the same as set forth in this schedule.

The rental of a room in hospital quarters would be optional on the part of the nurse and would not exceed $15.00 per month. The hospital could require the nurse to have her laundry done by the hospital laundry, but the charge for such service would not exceed $5.00 per month and was to include not less than three uniforms a week.

Hospitals and other institutions were to urge all members of nursing staffs to be members of the Michigan State Nurses Association and to require all members to be registered in Michigan.

The Ann Arbor District reported a record turn-out of 150 nurses for its October 16, 1945 meeting. This would have been the first meeting after the end of the war. Thelma Brewington, executive secretary of the Michigan State Nurses Association, was the speaker of the evening, and discussed Personnel Practices and

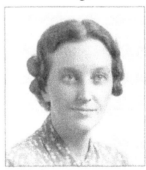

Policies for Michigan Nurses. Personnel practices and policies was the term used to describe the Association's work on improving the economic and working conditions of nurse members.

Thelma Brewington

Lulu St. Claire Blaine reported that more than 200 nurses attended the October 17 meeting of the Detroit District to hear a discussion of Personnel Employment Policies by Mrs. Edith Stamm, a staff nurse at Florence

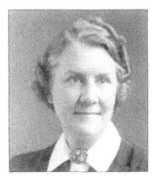

Lulu St. Claire Blaine

Crittenton Hospital. Thelma Brewington also reported on the work of the State Committee on Personnel Policies and asked for a favorable vote on the principle of granting authority to the Michigan State Nurses' Association to mediate for the nurses of Michigan in relation to personnel policies.

1944-1953

by Jess Merrill

Timeline

Immunizations Save Lives, Employment Shifts, and a Nurse Shortage Begins

A decade of urgency. World War II had ended along with the associated price controls and rationing that prevented free spending, the famous "Baby Boom" began with soldiers returning home from war, and the demand for housing skyrocketed. The "GI Bill" enabled soldiers to afford college and prepare themselves for new jobs in a robust economy. And the United States Bureau of the Census recognized nursing as a profession.

The Army needed nurses towards the end of World War II, and needed nurses badly. As described in the Michigan State Nurses Association magazine, *The Michigan Nurse*, in February 1945:

> "The Army Nurse Corps needs 10,000 additional nurses at once. This number may be increased to 20,000 if the need of the Service demands it. Every day during December, 1944, 1,000 sick and wounded service men reached this country for hospital care. The January rate may be higher. These men require and deserve the best nursing care. Fully 70% of the Army Nurse Corps has already been sent overseas; to send more would strip Army hospitals on this side of staff nurses desperately needed here. There are too few nurses, both overseas and at home. Army hospitals are operating with as few as one nurse to 26 beds, while the authorized ratio is one nurse to 15 beds (one to 12 beds overseas). The Navy Nurse Corps must prepare for staffing six new hospital ships to be commissioned in the next six months, and several new hospitals are going into operation, as well as fleet and base hospitals overseas. The Navy's total need is 2,500 nurses immediately."

At home in Michigan, over 2,000 nurses had entered America's Armed Forces for World War II. Fortunately, World War II ended shortly after the plea for help, and the urgent need for nurses in the military diminished. A nursing shortage persisted through the 1950s exacerbated by the Korean War.

Ensign Jane Louise Eldridge, RN

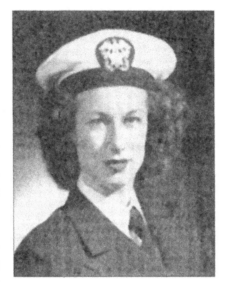

Ensign Jane Louise Eldridge, 28 years old, Navy Nurse Corps (Providence 1946) was the first Michigan nurse to be killed since the fighting in Korea began. With ten other nurses and other Navy personnel, she lost her life when their plane crashed in the Pacific on September 19, 1950.

A graduate of Northwestern High School, Detroit, Miss Eldridge had worked as a nurse's aide at Receiving Hospital before entering Providence Hospital School of Nursing in 1943, where she joined the U.S. Cadet Nurse Corps. While in school, according to faculty reports, "she distinguished herself by her diligent application to the task at hand, whether it was mastering her studies or acting as a hostess at a social function. Competent in all areas of nursing, she was well liked by her classmates and admired by her teachers."

After graduation she remained for a year as a staff nurse at Providence Hospital, living with her mother, Mrs. Lillian Eldridge, at 3287 Whitney Avenue, Detroit. She entered the Navy Nurse Corps in September 1947, and was stationed at the Naval Hospital, Bremerton, Washington. Here she made a rating of 97, the highest in her orientation class. She came home on leave September 2, 1950. Four days later her leave was cancelled, and she returned to Bremerton. Orders awaited her transferring her to the Naval Hospital at Yokosuka, Japan, where she would have become lieutenant, j.g. Ten other nurses went with her. On the way to Japan, the plane stopped for refuelling three times. When leaving the Kwajelein Islands after refuelling, the plane crashed in the ocean. All lives were lost.

The heartfelt sympathy of all Michigan nurses is extended to her mother.

Source: *The Michigan Nurse*, November 1950, pg. 148

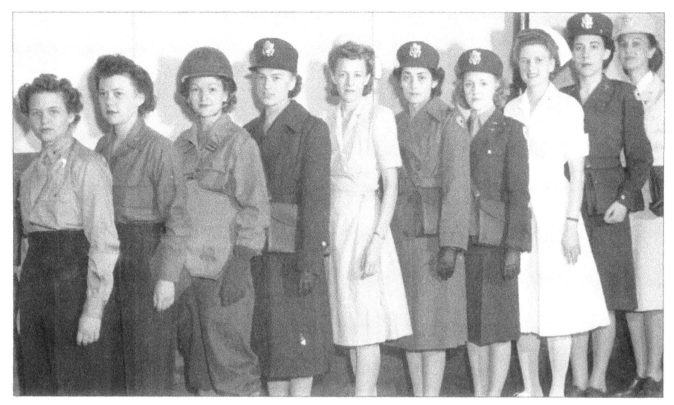

More than 2,000 Michigan nurses entered America's Armed Forces for World War II.

As the Michigan State Nurses Association entered its fourth decade, Association membership remained a concern. The MSNA Membership Committee expressed dismay over the loss of 17% of the Association's members from 1942-1944, and the Committee appealed to the district membership committees to respond to the loss of members. A plan was developed by the MSNA Membership Committee in January of 1945 that included the following suggestions for the district membership committees:

1. "Pep" letters could be written by the MSNA Committee and sent periodically from the office of the MSNA Executive Secretary to district membership committees, making suggestions and giving encouragement.

2. District membership committees should contact their schools of nursing and arrange to provide a speaker who could present the advantages of Association membership.

3. Membership and attendance at meetings depended upon interesting programs. The MSNA Executive Secretary could be contacted for program suggestions.

Along with the concern about Association membership was the work being done by the American Nurses Association, the National League of Nursing Education, and the National Organization for Public Health Nursing in ensuring the United States Bureau of the Census listed nurses as professionals when nurses identified their occupation for the Census. This work resulted in nurses being classified as "Professional and Technical Workers" in the Classified Index of Occupations during the 16th Census of the United States in 1940.

Chronic disease management continued as a primary activity of nurses. A general overview of successes in this area is reflected in an article in the October 1946 issue of *The Michigan Nurse*:

"Statistical results of efforts in which the Nursing Corps played so valiant a role were recently released by the Surgeon General's office. Comparative statistics of the four diseases causing the greatest loss of life in World Wars I and II are as follows:

Disease	World War I	World War II
Meningitis	38.0%	4.0%
Pneumonia	28.0%	0.7%
Tuberculosis	17.3%	2.0%
Dysentery	2.0%	<1.0%

Of course, many factors entered into the divergent results between these two wars. As might be expected, the tremendous achievements of the intervening 25 years in civilian practice were reflected in them. Affecting the total picture was the general immunization program for all personnel as part of their indoctrination and its continuance at proper intervals thereafter.

The development and thorough understanding of the use of the sulfonamide (sulfa drugs) group in the immediate pre-war years and the fortuitous appearance of penicillin in the early stages of the invasion of the continent played, undoubtedly, major roles in the insignificant mortalities of many previously highly lethal ailments. The use of whole blood or plasma early and in adequate quantities had an important share in lowering surgical mortalities, in particular; and on this score our wounded soldiers owe a profound debt of gratitude to the thousands of civilians who willingly gave their blood to this saving role."

Nurses' employment settings were changing. The October 1946 issue of *The Michigan Nurse* reports:

"A 1938 nationwide survey showed that of all graduates doing active nursing, 55% gave private duty as their principal occupation; 36% institutional nursing, and 9% Public Health. In 1943 over 60% were engaged in institutional nursing, approximately 10% each in public health and private duty nursing. [A remarkable change in 5 years!]

In 1945, 419 tuberculosis hospitals, with an average 175-bed capacity, reported less than 10 nurses per hospital, including all administrative branches. As of a few days ago, one such of our neighboring institutions, that at Northville, has 100 badly needed beds closed at present for lack of nurses, and only 49, instead of a normal 110 nurses, for the 715 patients there; while the State Sanatorium at Howell has 9 nurses for 385 patients."

Further chronic disease management concerns are reflected in *The Michigan Nurse*, June 1946, by Theodore J. Werle, Executive Secretary, Michigan Tuberculosis Association, who identified the paradox of empty beds and waiting lists.

"The problem facing Dr. Douglas, Detroit Health Commissioner, and others concerned with tuberculosis control are:

1) Michigan has a large number of tuberculous sick awaiting hospitalization; 2) several sanitoria have empty beds which the waiting patients could occupy; 3) an acute shortage of nurses prevents those beds from being used, so those on the waiting list continue to wait. Of the 4,686 existing beds, the Michigan Tuberculosis Association estimates about 700 are not in use."

MSNA remained committed to improving nurses' employment conditions, as reported in the January 1947 issue of *The Michigan Nurse*:

"Better employment conditions for nurses, secured through nurses' professional organizations are an essential step in providing better nursing service to the public, in the opinion of leaders of the American Nurses' Association [at the conclusion of] a three-day workshop on economic security."

Four Michigan nurses attended the ANA workshop on Economic Security: Kathleen Young, Hulda Erdman, Thelma Brewington and Winifred Kellogg.

"The conference, held at the Hamilton Hotel, brought together 70 representatives from 45 state nurses associations. Arranged by the ANA

Committee on Employment Conditions for Registered Nurses, it was designed to give practical help advancing the economic security program recommended by the national association for its 180,000 members at the biennial convention in Atlantic City, NJ, September, 1946.

Plans for action were based on the plank in the national platform calling for "improvement in hours and living conditions for nurses so that they may live a normal personal and professional life; wider acceptance of the 40-hour work week with no decrease in salary; and minimum salaries adequate to attract and hold nurses of quality and enable them to maintain standards of living comparable with other professions."

Collective bargaining as one means of reaching this goal is to be developed by many of the state nurses' associations, in line with the official policy stated as follows:

'The American Nurses Association believes that the several state and district nurses' associations are qualified to act and should act as the exclusive agents of their respective memberships in the important fields of economic security and collective bargaining. The Association commends the excellent progress already made and urges all state and district nurses' associations to push such a program vigorously and expeditiously.'

...Fact finding, standard setting, public education, and negotiations with employers are steps which most of the nurses' associations report they expect to take this winter.

State Nurses Associations were urged to do the following:

- Make the primary object of the program to assure the public of the quantity and quality of nursing service needed.

- Encourage nurses to set their own employment standards on a state-wide basis, through

sections of their state professional organization representing institutional staff nurses, those in private practice, public health, industry, etc.

- Know the state laws on labor relations and plan the nurses' program within that framework.

- Work out written agreements with individual institutions, such agreements to meet or exceed the state minimum.

- Use the technique of collective bargaining by the state nurses' professional organization when it seems advisable.

- Under no circumstances countenance a strike or similar coercive measures."

In 1947 Congress responded to labor unrest by passing the Labor-Management Relations Act, known as the Taft-Hartley Act, which placed limitations on the freedom to strike. The Taft-Hartley Act, passed over the veto of President Truman, was designed to roll back the gains made by labor during the New Deal. Known officially as the Labor-Management Relations Act, it was sponsored in the House by Fred Hartley, Jr., of New Jersey and in the Senate by Robert A. Taft of Ohio.

Its provisions made the closed shop illegal and outlawed secondary boycotts. Its most important provision gave the president the power to order a "cooling-off" period to stop strikes that threatened national safety or health. It also required unions to register and file financial reports with the Department of Labor, and union leaders had to swear under oath that they were not communists.

The Taft-Hartley Act hurt smaller unions, but the labor movement as a whole was not seriously weakened by the law. It did galvanize labor politically to battle Republicans in 1948, the year of Truman's upset victory over Thomas E. Dewey.

Nurses were once again called upon to support the nation's war efforts. By the end of 1950, 249 Army Nurse Corps officers were in Korea. The demand for more Army nurses in the combat zone drastically

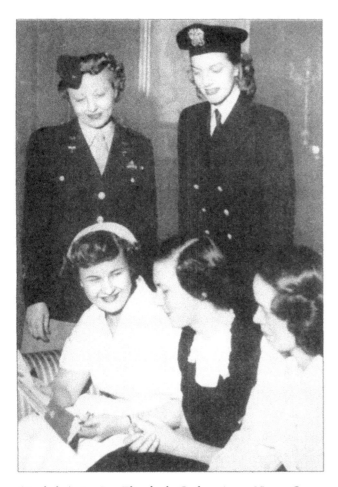

(Back l-r) 1st Lt. Elizabeth Cosler, Army Nurse Corps, and Lt. Lavinia Nyhuis, Nurse Corps, US Navy, were guest speakers at a meeting of the Detroit Inter Council of Future Nurses Clubs. (Front l-r) Past Club President and freshman student nurse Sally Thistle, President Phyllis Weeks and Secretary Betty Woods.

depleted nurse strength in other Army units worldwide. Additional Army Nurse Corps officers or even replacements were few as both the Army and the nation were in the midst of a nursing shortage dating back to 1945 and the end of World War II.

The exact number of Army Nurse Corps officers who saw action in the Korean War over the course of the three-year conflict is unknown; estimates vary from more than 500 to approximately 1,500. While not physically located in the combat zone, these women suffered many of the same deprivations, rose to meet similar relentless challenges and worked long, hard hours. The contributions of Army Nurse Corps officers who served during the Korean War were significant.

At the close of this decade, there were 6,913 members and 40 district associations in the Michigan State Nurses Association. Tri-County had disbanded into the original districts of Delta, Dickenson, and Menominee, and Oceana and Muskegon districts were again separate entities. There were 74 individual members scattered throughout the state.

Nurses were urged to join or renew their memberships through the district association except in those areas where there was no organized district association. Dues for an active nurse were $13.25, plus district dues which varied. Associate members (those engaged in the practice of nursing fewer than 30 days per year) paid to the state office a total of $2.75 for which they received *The Michigan Nurse,* but were ineligible to participate in group rates for Blue Cross, or Group Sickness and Accident Insurance.

CHAPTER 6

1954-1963

by Jess Merrill

Timeline

1954 –50th anniversary year; 40 districts now constituents of MNSA

1955 – Industrial Nurses Branch of MSNA formed

1956 – MSNA urged nurses to participate in civil defense preparation; increased MSNA state dues to $10.00

1957 – The optimum ratio was 300 RNs per 100,000 persons in the general population; 70,000 more nurses needed to meet that goal

1958 – Annual convention included the first House of Delegates; Economic Security Program (ESP) was created

1959 – The *American Journal of Nursing* added as a membership benefit; MSNA stood at 51 districts; MSNA supported the Landrum-Griffin Act

1960 – Economic security a top priority

1961 – MSNA developed first legislative platform; ANA called for amendment to Taft-Hartley; MSNA began to study nurses' salaries by areas of Michigan

1962 – JFK appointed committee to study nursing shortage; Governor's Commission formulated 45 recommendations for nursing

1963 – Members collected Green Stamps for a new building; MSNA changed to MNA at convention

Civil Defense Nursing and Low Wages; Nurses Organize for Economic Security

Disputes between the Soviet Union and the Western democracies led to a long period of East-West tension and conflict that became known as the "Cold War." It was characterized by mutual perceptions of hostile intent between the East and West, and each side amassed huge stockpiles of nuclear weapons.

The United States was under the leadership of President Dwight D. Eisenhower until John F. Kennedy became the youngest and first Catholic president in 1961. Less than three years into his presidency, he was shot to death while riding in a motorcade in Dallas, Texas. The nation reeled in shock as the new techology of television brought the tragedy directly into their living rooms. Vice President Lyndon Johnson then assumed the role of president and was elected for another term.

In this context, MSNA marked its 50th year. A variety of anniversary tributes were included in *The Michigan Nurse* during this year. The Executive Secretary of MNSA's Detroit District wrote this editorial:

"A great many Americans have a very high regard for the women performing nursing services. We pay grateful tribute to the war effort of the nursing profession. Yet many Americans believe there is room for improvement in the performances of nurses in present-day hospital and private practice, especially in public health and industrial nursing. There is a general belief that the cost of nursing is too high.

The *American Journal of Nursing* says that these findings lead the way to some conclusions and recommendations. It has been found that the nursing profession is a desirable one, but offers too little recompense to those who practice it and is offered at too high a charge to those who need it…Those two contradictions must be resolved by changes in the present method of distributing and paying for nursing services, changes which will serve to raise salaries and yet lower costs to the public."

Michigan Nurses Week, 1954

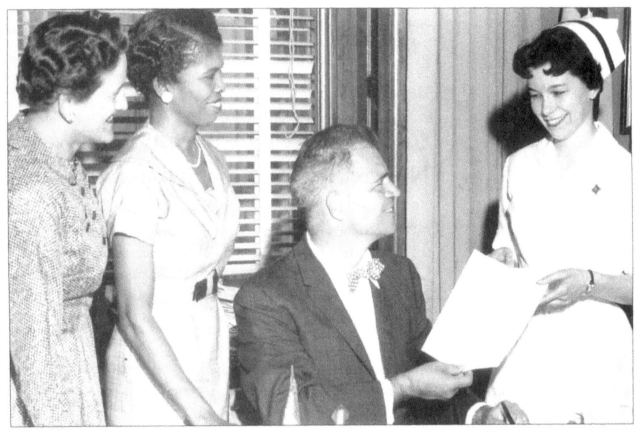

During MSNA's Golden Anniversary year, Governor G. Mennen Williams signed the proclamation of Michigan Nurses Week which paid tribute to to the pioneer nurses and those who follow in their footsteps.

This year, on the fiftieth anniversary of the founding of the State Nurses Association, more than 7,000 professional nurses, now practicing in Michigan under provisions of [the Licensure and Registration Act], will honor with appropriate ceremonies the courageous women to whose efforts, half a century ago, they are so profoundly indebted for the benefits which they enjoy today.

Therefore, I, G. Mennen Williams, Governor of the State of Michigan, do hereby proclaim the period from May 9 through May 15, 1954, which includes the Golden Anniversary of the Michigan State Nurses Association, as

MICHIGAN NURSES WEEK

and urge all our citizens during this week to join in paying tribute not only to the pioneer nurses of our state but to all who follow the nursing profession and who, with each advance in the art of healing, are contributing in ever greater measure to the health and welfare of our state and nation.

Signed the fifth day of April,
in the year of Our Lord, One thousand nine hundred fifty-four,
and of the Commonwealth, the One hundred eighteenth.
G. Mennen Williams, Governor

As MSNA celebrated its golden anniversary in 1954, African American nurses were not part of its history. African American nurses were not allowed to be ANA members until 1951 when members of the National Association of Colored Graduate Nurses (NACGN) were successful in their demand for change.

A guest editorial in the May 9, 1954 *Lansing State Journal* by Florence Kempf, RN, entitled "Nursing in 1904, 1954, and Beyond" describes what an individual nurse believed at the time of MSNA's 50th year.

"…The professional nurses in Michigan can take justifiable pride in the developments and contributions of their organization. They cannot, however, meditate long on what has gone before because urgent nursing demands require that, as stock taking goes on, attention must be focused on the goals for the future.

How can the Michigan State Nurses Association better serve its members and in the process contribute more surely to the health of Michigan? Nursing is one of the social forces that functions to serve mankind, and, so doing, participates in the building of a better world."

During the last year the Cunningham Drug Foundation financed a survey of needs and resources 'For Better Nursing in Michigan,' which was sponsored by the Michigan State Nurses Association and others.

Briefly, the study shows that there is a shortage of professional nurses employed in Michigan; the distribution of those who are available further complicates the picture. Our general hospitals caring for less than half of Michigan's ill employ about 90 percent of the professional nurses and almost 50 percent of the non-nurse personnel, while our tuberculosis and mental hospitals caring for more than one-half of Michigan's patients employ less than 10 percent of the professional nurses and 33 percent of the non-nurse personnel.

This survey points the way to action, not only to all nurses in Michigan but to all community groups and leaders that are concerned with improvement in the care of patients and in the health of our citizens. We, in Michigan, are fortunate to have the problems which confront us so clearly defined; and working together we can effect the changes that eventually will bring better nursing to Michigan."

In response to the Cold War, a nation-wide Civil Defense plan was initiated, managed by the individual states, and implemented at the local level. Part of the plan was to train nurses on the aspects of atomic warfare. Michigan nurses responded, as evidenced in the June 1955 issue of *The Michigan Nurse* article written by Jean E. Jeffries, RN, who was the coordinator of the Wayne Joint Committee for nursing in civic defense. The article was entitled "Who Needs Civic Defense" and brings to mind today, bioterrorism training.

"The answer is that *you* do…to be of service to anyone else, every nurse must first know how to care for herself and for her family. She must be informed on the latest civil defense developments, and the activity of the local, state, and federal civil defense organizations.

The advent of the hydrogen bomb has made [civil defense] a problem for us all. Radioactive fall-out will not be confined to the target area. Large numbers of people on the move will create public health problems and, rest assured, the people from the cities will be moving to rural areas whether the community is prepared or not.

The threat is real; the enemy has the bombs as well as the means of delivering them. What better antidote for fear than to be actively engaged in civil defense, the most important civic project to date. As in any other cooperative effort, the rewards can be satisfying."

In a June 1955 letter to *The Michigan Nurse* editor, Eileen Poyer, RN, District Nurses Civil Defense Chairman for Calhoun County asks:

"Do we have a State Director of Nursing in Civil Defense? Is there a state civil defense plan as yet and what is the nurse's part in it as far Michigan is concerned? Is there a specific Civil Defense act of legislation in Michigan concerning the practice of nursing and duties [a nurse] may be expected to assume in an emergency? Is there a state manual guide for nursing? What are nurses doing elsewhere in the state?"

In response Isabelle Ryer, RN, Chairman, Michigan State Committee on Nursing in National Defense, wrote:

"Dear Mrs. Poyer:

You ask is there a State Director of Nursing in Civil Defense – the answer is yes and no. The Federal Civil Defense Act of 1950, Public Law 920 gives the responsibility to the states 'for providing leadership and supervision in civil defense planning within their boundaries.'

The State Health Commissioner is charged with the responsibility for providing a plan for health services and medical care in the event of a military disaster. It follows that the Director of Nursing Service in the State Health Department would, in effect, be responsible for nursing in civil defense. The latter is not clearly stated, but rather assumed. Further, the nurse's role is not separately outlined in the civil defense plan, but rather integrated in terms of teams and areas of assignment of these teams.

Regarding a manual: the only document, which the nurses in Michigan have prepared on this subject, is the manual, *Suggested Course of Study for Graduate Nurses in Medical and Nursing Aspects of Atomic Warfare*. There is a manual issued by the Federal Civil Defense Administration, TM 11-7, *The Nurse in Civil Defense*.

No doubt you know that the Detroit medical plan is probably the most developed of any in the state. Casualty stations have been established,

training courses have been instituted, meetings of the casualty care teams are held regularly and a test run was carried out last November."

As the fear of the Cold War subsided, the Michigan State Nurses Association resumed its focus on internal issues such as an economic security program.

The necessity of the Economic Security Program was emphasized in June 1957 when the Bureau of Labor Statistics released information that showed the weekly salaries of nurses employed in some of the country's major cities. Nurses in Chicago hospitals averaged $73 for general duty nurses to $119 for nursing directors. The highest paid chief X-ray technicians earned $86.50, whereas X-ray technicians and medical technologists earned $70 and $71 respectively. In St. Louis nurses earned $66 a week, head nurses $74 a week and instructors $74.50 a week. In Boston staff nurses averaged $64.50 and directors of nursing $100.50 a week. Hospitals in Cincinnati and Boston paid similar salaries to their nurses.

At the annual meeting in October 1958, the members of the Michigan State Nurses Association voted to adopt an Economic Security Program (ESP) for the organization. The ESP Committee was established in December, 1958 and reappointed in 1959 with Mary Weinschreider, RN, as its able chairwoman.

The Board of Directors endorsed the program as vital for the organization and created a professional staff position filled by Miss Avis Dykstra, RN who joined the association as Assistant Executive Director on April 25, 1959. Mrs. Kay Fuller and Daniel H. Kruger, PhD were retained as consultants in public and industrial relations.

The main purpose of the ESP was to improve employment conditions for nurses and to relate the program to other activities of the association. The board regarded it as essential in achieving the objectives of the organization – the provision of quality nursing care.

Avis J. Dykstra, RN, highlights how the ESP was working in the May/June 1959 edition of *The Michigan Nurse*:

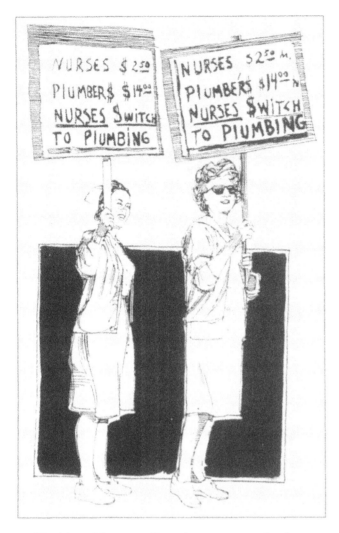

"In this article we are featuring an approach where the professional staff nurses work with a MSNA representative to obtain improved employment conditions.

In all, there are about 100 professional nurses on the staff of Pontiac General Hospital. Sixty-six percent of them are MSNA members and pay $25.50 yearly dues for membership in their professional association and refuse to become unionized.

The hospital administration has recognized MSNA as the official representative agent for the professional nursing staff and has had the opportunity to interpret some of their problems and obstacles in making changes.

The nurses from Pontiac General hospital feel that this cooperative approach in working toward improved employment practices has been very

rewarding. We feel that strong progress has been made and that the hospital's nurses have truly benefited from their participation in this program.

This is a good example of how nurses can – and do – have a voice in determining their own employment conditions."

In *The Michigan Nurse*, September/October 1962 issue, further progress of the Economic Security Program is noted:

"During the past year MSNA has officially represented nurses to their employer in seven hospitals and three health departments.

…professional standards and economic security do go 'hand-in-hand." Every professional nurse should make it her business to improve professional practice through improved conditions of employment."

Luther Christman, RN, MSNA President, writes in the same issue:

"The American Nurses' Association unequivocally opposes strikes among nurses.

But 'mass resignations' by nurses is a different matter. The association has not as yet taken an official stand on such a procedure.

Speaking personally, and not as a spokesman for any official group, I feel that mass resignations are perfectly legitimate.

…At a small Illinois hospital mass resignations occurred this year. After fruitless attempts at negotiation with hospital administrators, the nurses finally decided to stage mass resignations. These resignations were staggered in such a way that hospital administrators would have ample time to recruit qualified replacements.

As a direct outcome of the mass resignations, salaries at this hospital were substantially increased, working conditions were improved, and new equipment was obtained. In short, the net result was better patient care."

As has been part of the Association's history, partnerships with legislators were vital in advancing nursing's agenda.

Congressman James G. O'Hara (D-Michigan 7th District), presented a paper at the ANA Convention, Detroit, Michigan, May 15, 1962, in which he stated:

"…In charting the legislative actions needed to improve the professional security of nurses, a history book is a more useful instrument than a compass.

Nurses have the same problems as other employed persons. They need income protection for periods of retirement, disability and involuntary unemployment. They need an income commensurate with their training, skill and responsibility. They have a right to participate in decisions affecting their compensation, their working conditions and the nursing practices of the institution in which they are employed.

…Happily, the Kennedy administration has demonstrated an awareness of this problem and has already asked Congress to set standards, which would, among other things, extend unemployment compensation coverage to non-profit organizations including hospitals.

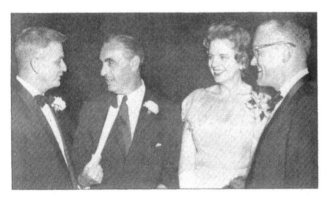

MNA President Luther Christman, RN (far left) and Congressman James G. O'Hara (D-Utica) (far right), brief the Honorable Abraham Ribicoff, Secretary of Health, Education and Welfare and ANA President Margaret B. Dolan, RN, on the local situation following the Secretary's opening address to the ANA's 42nd biennial convention.

I am firmly of the belief that removal of the hospital exemption from the Fair Labor Standards Act should be one of the legislative goals of the ANA. It should be so for two reasons.

First, studies of ANA and the Bureau of Labor Statistics have demonstrated that a significant amount of employment in excess of 40 hours per week still exists in nursing and that most nurses working more than 40 hours a week do not receive time and half for hours in excess of 40 as required by the Fair Labor Standards Act.

Secondly, and even more importantly, nurse's salaries have lagged seriously behind those of other professionals performing work requiring a comparable degree of ability, skill and responsibility. This explains, to a large extent, the continuing shortage of registered nurses."

In 1959 Congress passed the Landrum-Griffin Act, officially known as the Labor-Management Reporting and Disclosure Act (LMRDA). The purpose of the Act was to provide for the reporting and disclosure of certain financial transactions and administrative practices of labor organizations and employers, to provide standards with respect to the election of officers of labor organizations, and for other purposes.

Hyman Parker, LLB, Hearings Officer for the Michigan State Labor Mediation Board, delivered a presentation at the 1961 MSNA Convention on current labor laws. Excerpts from his remarks follow:

"In a recent publication, the American Hospital Association recognized the following trend: 'It is anticipated that Unions will make further efforts in the near future to obtain a greater number of members among hospital employees.'

A 1959 survey by the Michigan Hospital Association showed, among other things, that only two hospitals reported "unionization" of practical nurses, registered nurses, and X-ray technicians.

The American Nurses' Association in implementing its 'Economic Security Program' at its

1958 national convention passed a resolution to take "immediate steps to implement in all hospitals the essential practices of collective bargaining:

1. Freedom of employees to organize.

2. Free choice of representation.

3. Recognition of employees' representatives and bargaining in good faith by representatives of employers and employees.

4. Negotiations and signed contracts

By 1958, registered nurses in seven states had contracts with 87 hospitals. In 1960, six state nurses' associations had agreements with 120 institutions covering approximately 8,000 registered professional nurses."

Membership in MSNA remained an issue of discussion. Lystra Gretter, Lulu Cudney, Emilie Sargent, Grace Ross, Lulu St. Clair Blaine, and other charter members and their successors considered membership in the professional association as an obligation of the practitioner, and those serious about the profession of nursing would, of course, become a member of the Michigan State Nurses Association.

An article stressing the benefits and importance of membership appeared in the January 1958 issue of *The Michigan Nurse*:

"What does the Michigan State Nurses Association do for me? Why should I belong? These are familiar questions. Let us review some of the activities of our Association to help answer them for you.

The MNSA, since its origin in 1904, has directed its activities toward the following objectives: continuing improvement in nursing practice, in the welfare of nurses, and in health care of the people. Through membership in the professional association, each nurse supports the programs designed to further these objectives.

Some activities benefit the nurse directly, some indirectly by strengthening the nursing profession.

Some activities of the Michigan State Nurses Association are as follows:

1. MAINTAINS a central headquarters office.

2. CONDUCTS the business activities of the Association through personal contacts and correspondence.

3. PROVIDES AND CONDUCTS a Professional Counseling and Placement Service.

4. PROMOTES legislation and speaks for nurses and nursing in regard to legislative action concerning general health and welfare programs.

5. SUPPORTS efforts of the ANA to secure federal legislation.

6. MAKES AVAILABLE to its members various types of group insurance.

7. PREPARES AND PUBLISHES recommended personnel policies for the various sections of the Association.

8. PUBLISHES *The Michigan Nurse* and distributes other information to its members.

9. HOLDS annual meetings to conduct the business of the Association and to provide programs of interest and benefit to nurses.

10. SERVES as a clearing house for scheduling conferences, workshops and meetings sponsored by various agencies, for nurses and nursing groups.

11. REIMBURSES expenses incurred when members attend MSNA board or committee meetings.

12. WORKS jointly with other organizations in presenting educational programs and information to nurses.

13. STUDIES nursing needs and resources in Michigan.

14. PARTICIPATES in plans with hospital, medical allied professional groups, and

voluntary associations for the improvement of patient care.

15. PROMOTES and co-sponsors with the Michigan League for Nursing the Michigan State Student Nurses Association.

16. ENDEAVORS to promote equal educational and employment opportunities for all nurses regardless of race or creed.

17. IMPLEMENTS the international exchange of nurses program; provides observation and training experiences for foreign nurses.

18. PROVIDES through the MSNA Service Fund, a small temporary stipend for sick and needy nurses.

19. MAKES AVAILABLE services of legal counsel on professional problems through the MSNA headquarters office.

20. REPRESENTS and serves nurses as their official spokesman with allied professional and governmental groups and with the public.

MSNA is your organization and its strength is measured by the contribution of the individual nurses. I belong…do you?"

A nursing shortage existed throughout WWII and became critical in the early 1960s, as reported in the July/August 1961 issue of *The Michigan Nurse*:

"While the reported 35% shortage at Detroit Receiving is acute, so are shortages in other hospitals throughout the city which have as much as 30% and more of their budgeted nursing positions unfilled. The problem is not isolated – it is an around the clock, year-in and year-out situation which promises only to get worse.

In the greater Detroit area, as a whole, twenty percent of the budgeted nursing positions in hospitals remain vacant. State-wide there is a 16% shortage of hospital nurses.

Why? This is generally the first question asked by the layman and often by nurses themselves.

Unfortunately, we don't have all the answers, but we can and do point out that the average general duty hospital nurse in Michigan earns $79.00 a week, and $85.00 a week in the Detroit area. This doesn't compare very favorably with typists, accounting clerks, secretaries and tabulating machine operators in Detroit who average from $89.50 to $114.50 a week."

In the same issue, it was noted that President Kennedy appointed a committee to study the nursing shortage.

"The nursing profession is already facing an acute shortage, and the demand for augmented and new services essential for an adequate health program promises to grow. The advice of physicians, hospital administrators, nurses, educators, social scientists, and public health executives is being sought to help devise a program that will meet the needs of the nation.

Secretary Abraham Ribicoff told the Surgeon General's Consultant Group on Nursing, at their first meeting in Washington…that the nurse is the 'magic ingredient in health services.'

As a preliminary step, the group proposes to explore the social, economic and scientific developments which have accelerated demands on nursing, conditions of supply and demand in the various nursing fields, and types of programs which prepare personnel for careers in nursing. It is expected to consider specific problems encountered in the practice of nursing which are not faced in the practice of other professions. A most important concern is the part the Federal government should take in the support of nursing education."

A few novel issues captured the attention of the Association as it completed its sixth decade. These included a new headquarters building, a name change, and future concerns. The following excerpts from *The Michigan Nurse* highlight these issues.

"Our Site's in Sight" (from *The Michigan Nurse*, May/June 1963) – "At last it's out. The MSNA

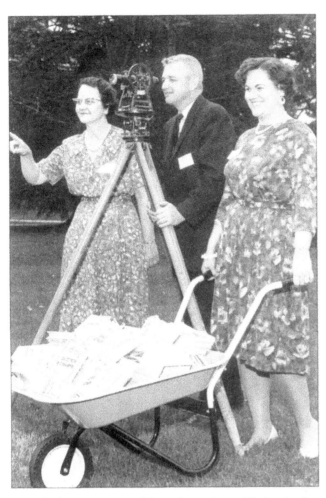

Elizabeth Vigeant, Building Committee Chair; Luther Christman, president, and Eleanor Tromp, Executive Secretary set their sights on a new headquarters building.

Green Stamp campaign is a project of the Building Committee to buy land for a building site. Representatives from the Sperry and Hutchinson Green Stamp Company are intrigued with the suggestion to convert stamps to money in order to purchase land."

"Why a Name Change?" (from *The Michigan Nurse,* July/August 1963) – "With the proposed revision of the Nursing Practice Act, reference is made in the context of this bill to the Michigan Nurses Association. If we do not change our

name and permit the bill to go to legislature as it is, there is the possibility that the bill would then need to be reopened for this modified change. We are hopeful that the House of Delegates will approve of the name change and eliminate the need for any further amending of the Nursing Practice Act."

And lastly, as MNA approached a new decade, President Luther Christman, RN, identified issues that are relevant today:

"From the President's Desk," *The Michigan Nurse,* January/February 1964 – "Three of the many issues facing the organization stand out with remarkable clarity.

A burning and primary issue is the need to close the economic gap between present salary levels paid to nurses and those paid to other professional groups with comparative training.

A second gnawing problem is that of MNA district structure. Do we have too many (51) districts? Should minimum standards as to membership size and operations processes be established? Are we weakened by being splintered into segments too small for constructive action?

A third issue is one of setting priorities for organizational activity. Which of the many programs now being conducted or in the planning stage should have priority? What programs should have the concentration of staff and committee activity? With limited resources – both of staff and money – where should we invest these resources for the greatest professional gain?"

Those Who Marched
Luther Christman, RN, PhD, FAAN

by Jess Merrill

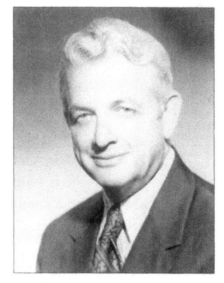

Luther Christman wanted a career that he and his wife-to-be could enjoy together. They both enrolled in nursing schools in Philadelphia – Luther in the Pennsylvania School of Nursing for Men, and Dorothy in the Methodist Hospital School of Nursing.

Luther was just beginning his career when World War II began. At the time male nurses were not allowed to serve in their chosen profession and he spent the greater part of his military career as a pharmacist's mate in the US Maritime Service. After the war Luther returned to Pennsylvania Hospital where he worked as a private duty nurse and assistant head nurse.

In 1948 he received a BSN at Temple University, and in 1952 completed a master's degree in educational psychology. He began developing his belief that entrance into the profession should be at an advanced degree level. From 1953-1956 Luther worked as director of nursing at Yankton State Hospital in Yankton, South Dakota.

When he became a nurse consultant for the State of Michigan's Department of Mental Health in 1956, he became very active in the Michigan Nurses Association. Elected as MNA's first male president in 1961, he was re-elected in 1963. He was also accepted at Michigan State University as a doctoral candidate in sociology and anthropology.

He accepted a position as associate professor of psychiatric nursing at the University of Michigan in 1963, during his second term as MNA president.

At the ANA Convention in 1964, Luther proposed the establishment of the American Academy of Nursing. His resolution was overwhelmingly passed by the House of Delegates. The Academy was not, however, implemented until 1973 when ANA named 36 charter fellows as pro-tem officers. Luther was inducted into the Academy in 1974.

In 1967 Luther accepted a position as dean of nursing at Vanderbilt University in Nashville, Tennessee. It was the first time a man had been named dean of a university school of nursing.

Luther moved to Rush University, Chicago in 1972 where he became very influential in placing the practitioner/teacher model into effect. The emphasis was on education from the undergraduate level to doctorally prepared nurses. Clinical practice, teaching, research, and consultation were all elements of the program.

He was instrumental in establishing the American Assembly of Men in Nursing in 1971, and he served as its permanent chairman while at Rush.

Dr. Luther Christman is well known around the globe for his controversial ideas regarding advanced degree requirements for entry into the profession, and for his notion that if the majority of American nurses had been men, the economic and general welfare of nurses would never have been an issue.

1964-1973

by Carol Feuss

Social Unrest; Nurses Fight for Equality and Acceptance of Nursing Practice Act

This was the decade of social unrest, when both people and systems were being redefined, often violently. When assassinations took the lives of Dr. Martin Luther King, Jr., a strong leader in the Civil Rights movement and Senator Robert Kennedy, people struggled to find balance in a country already caught up in a war overseas. The passing of the Civil Rights Act in 1964 forced schools to become integrated almost overnight while groups such as the militant Black Panther Party for Self-Defense tried to protect minority communities from interference by the government. In April of 1965, President Johnson authorized the use of ground combat troops for offensive action in Vietnam, and the face of US universities changed as an era of anti-war protests began. At the height of the protests in 1970, tragedy struck as four students were killed and eight injured at Kent State University in Ohio. Fueled by an already tense atmosphere, 75,000 students gathered in Washington, DC in a volatile anti-war demonstration.

Even though these were turbulent times, great strides were being made in technology and science. This expertise enabled the landing of Apollo 11 on the moon, the launching of the Internet, the arrival of word processing machines in offices, and the founding of Microsoft. In healthcare the first successful human heart transplant was performed, war was declared on cancer, abortion was legalized, and the Occupational Health and Safety Act was passed. The advent of Medicare was established in 1965 through amendments to the Social Security Act. MNA's seventh decade came to a close with the resignation of President Richard Nixon.

By the time American troops withdrew from Vietnam in 1974, almost 6,000 nurses and medical specialists had been deployed. The Vietnam nurses memorial in Washington, DC stands as a testimony to those who served in those horrific times, providing care and compassion with honor and strength.

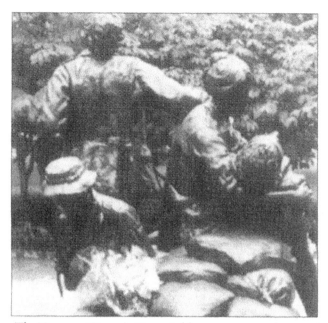

The Vietnam Women's Memorial honors women who served in the military during the Vietnam War.

Never straying far from its beginnings and reflecting the changing times, the mid '60s saw MNA advocating for the nursing profession, but in new ways.

Strengthening the practice of nursing through education was a major theme in the mid '60s:

> "Five MNA goals…are directly related to education for nurses: basic and continuing education for nursing practice, refresher courses for inactive nurses, and leadership training for MNA members to strengthen the effectiveness of the association."

The debate centering on "entry into practice" grew more vocal during this time. Following the American Nurses Association lead, MNA went on record in 1964 as supporting the belief that:

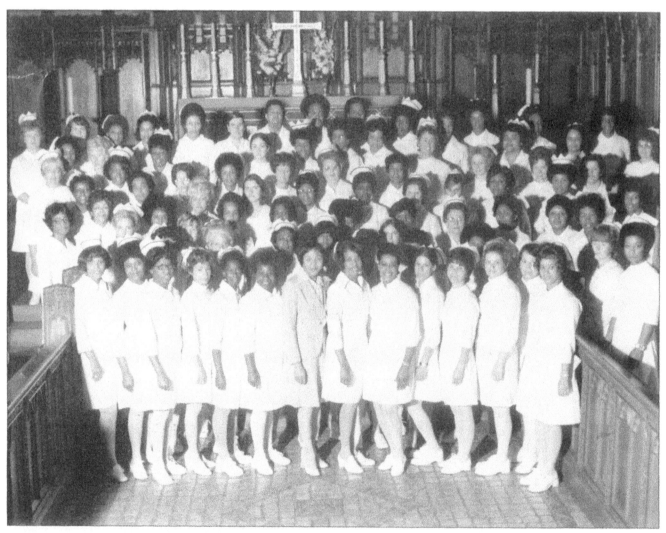

First graduates from the Associate Degree Program at Wayne County Community College (May 1972).

"technical and professional education should be the basic preparation for nursing. To this end, the preparation of nurse technicians and the preparation of professional nurses should be in institutions of higher learning."

In September 1965 there were six baccalaureate degree programs, ten associate degree programs and 21 diploma programs in Michigan.

During this time, MNA pushed for the Nursing Practice Act, first introduced in 1965 as Senate Bill 19. MNA President Luther Christman testified to the State Affairs Committee in support of this bill:

"We believe this bill will protect the public from untrained personnel and help to insure safe nursing practices...In order to clarify the roles, it is suggested that only two groups in nursing be licensed – registered nurses (RN) and licensed practical nurse (LPN)...The definition of practice as a registered nurse [includes]:...1) supervision of the patient involving the whole management of his nursing care; 2) the observation of symptoms and reactions both physical and mental; 3) the accurate recording and reporting of facts including evaluation of total care; 4) supervision and teaching of other personnel; 5) the carrying out of nursing procedures and techniques; 6) the maintenance of health and prevention of illness of others; and 7) the administration of medications and treatments prescribed by a licensed physician or dentist."

At their spring meeting in1966 the MNA Board

"decided that MNA will not introduce any nursing practice act legislation at this time since the association does not have the firm support and commitment of all nursing groups."

However, the bill was reintroduced in 1966, without MNA's backing.

Christman noted:

"One can become very battered and groggy struggling against the waves of change but can experience a tingling exuberance riding the crest of change. Riding these waves of change can be in the fashion of the clumsy canoeist who capsizes the craft or in the manner of the skillful surfer who plots his course to take maximum advantage of surf and current. The delicate art of assuring one's destiny is worth all the time, effort, and professional talent available to the profession."

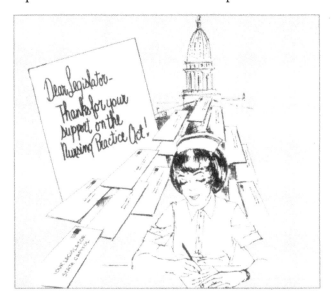

The Nursing Practice Act, signed into law in 1967, clarified licensure and defined the role of the nurse.

June 30, 1967 saw a new Nursing Practice Act bill introduced, passed, and signed into law by Governor Romney. The Act would change nursing in Michigan forever, as RNs gained the ability to practice without being under the direction of another person.

As the legislative dispute for the Nursing Practice Act was ongoing, other legislation passed that altered the face of health care:

1) Michigan Labor Mediation Act (Act No 176 of the Public Acts of 1939 as amended, formerly called the Bonine Tripp Act) gave employees of *private* agencies the right to organize and bargain collectively with their employers.

2) Public Employment Relations Act (Act No 336 of the Public Acts of 1947 as amended, formerly called the Hutchinson Act) gave employees of *public* agencies the right to organize and bargain collectively with their employers.

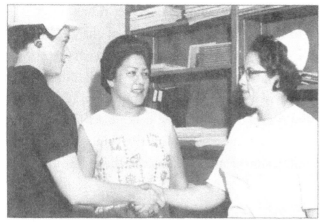

MNA President Jessie Pergrin, RN (l) welcomes Mattie Williams, RN, a new nurse at Metropolitan Hospital, to Michigan. Watching is Mrs. Ursula Somera, RN, Metropolitan Hospital's Director of Nursing.

As Jessie V. Pergrin, RN, of the Greater Detroit district, became President in 1965, MNA had been providing "ESP consultation" for almost seven years.

These two acts changed MNA's relationship with hospitals, as noted in a 1966 letter from MNA President Jessie V. Pergrin, RN, to the Directors of Nursing in Michigan hospitals:

"The recent MNA Convention considered the situation at considerable length and the House of Delegates' conclusion was to authorize MNA to act as a collective bargaining representative for groups of registered nurses when the nurses in a given employing unit request it."

Nurses were quick to respond to this new opportunity, as the MNA Staff 1966 Convention Annual report notes:

"For the first time, some employers have recognized the MNA as the exclusive bargaining representative of registered nurses." In the first year these nurses in public institutions were represented under Public Act 379: Dickinson County Hospitals, Iron Mountain – MNA recognized by election; County of Wayne (Health Department and Hospitals) – voluntary recognition; Alpena General Hospital – voluntary recognition; City of Flint Department of Public Health – voluntary recognition; Highland Park

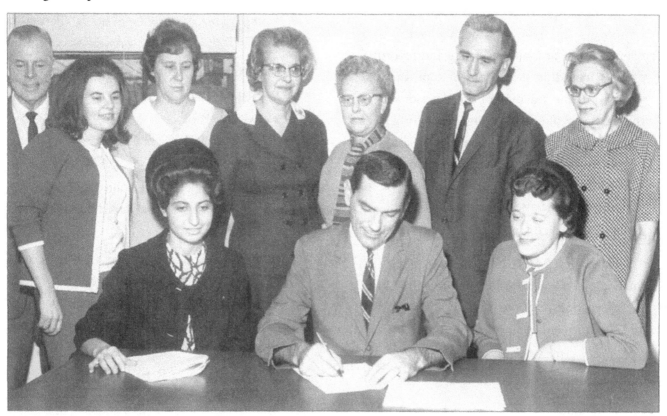

MNA officials sign the State's first RN Labor Agreement at Highland Park General Hospital. It calls for salary increases from 10 to 13% for staff nurses and "elimination of MOST dietary, housekeeping and pharmacy functions from the nursing department" and, an "allowance of up to $250 a year for further study."

General Hospital – voluntary recognition; and City of Detroit – recognition pending.

The Michigan Nurse stated, "The staff council at Little Traverse Hospital in Petoskey was the first in the state to conduct economic security negotiations in a private institution." Their reason for organizing, as explained by staff council chair Mrs. Kathleen Vander Weele, RN, rings true today:

> "Our staff council was organized because of the prevalence of low and inequitable salaries, poor delineation of job classifications, outmoded personnel policies, and increasingly low morale of professional workers. The need for an organization backed by MNA was apparent when individuals and small groups were unable to correct these conditions by appeals to the hospital administrator through proper channels."

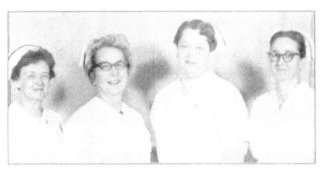

Negotiating Committee members from Little Traverse Hospital (l-r): Mrs. M. Katherine Worthen, RN, treasurer; Mrs. Kathleen Vander Weele, RN, president; Faye Pitman, RN, vice president; and Ruth Culp, RN, secretary.

In 1967, there were 32 such groups of nurses who sought MNA assistance and received ESP consultation. The ESP program was now seen as a way to increase membership: "Most of the RNs in a particular facility or location must belong to MNA before MNA can undertake specific or detailed ESP assistance."

With a growing emphasis on economic issues, Gene Malis joined MNA's staff to "negotiate nurse contracts throughout the state" and Daniel Kruger, PhD was the ESP consultant. In 1967 MNA contracted with Industrial Relations Staff Services to provide ESP consultation.

The MNA Board of Directors voted at their April 25, 1968 meeting to create a separate Economic Security Program and appointed Eleanor M. Tromp, RN, as executive director of the new ESP organization while looking for a director. The steering committee for ESP was named as the interim board of directors, until October, 1968.

An organizational meeting was held on October 29, at the Sheraton-Cadillac Hotel in Detroit. Bylaws and new officers were elected. Eleanor M. Tromp, RN, MNESO Executive Administrator and Eugene Malis, MNESO Staff report in 1969:

> "MNA announced the arrived of a 'blessed event' in October 1968 – the new Division MNESO – Michigan Nurses Economic Security Organization). This division was created within MNA to more effectively represent the economic interests of our members. Conflict of interest was inherent on the MNA Board of Directors before the creation of MNESO. At that time the sixteen-member MNA Board of Directors had representation of nine nursing administrators or over 50 per cent."

In 1968, PASS (Professional Association Staff Services) of Detroit had the contract to negotiate

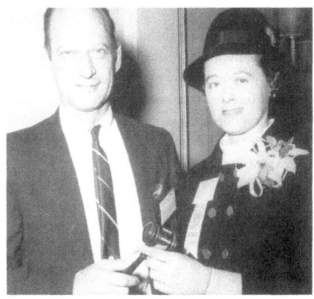

President John H. Wick, RN accepts the MNA gavel from immediate Past-President Jessie V. Pergrin, RN at the 1967 MNA convention.

agreements on behalf of MNESO. In 1969, MNA employed two new negotiators Miss Mary Ellen Trottner and Mr. Larry Bishop "…with the goal to gradually phase out the consulting firm." The relationship with PASS turned bitter in 1970 as they filed an Unfair Labor Practice against MNA on behalf of 45 nurses, and MNA brought a civil suit against PASS. Much time and resources were spent on this conflict, but it reinforced the need for the separation between the MNA board and the ESP program.

In 1971, the MNA ESP staff was in its first full year of operation and the first "Council on Economic and General Welfare" was elected:

Ruth DeNeff, RN (Ottawa) (PHN)
Eileen Williams, RN (Bay) (GDN)
Ruby Merkle, RN (Branch-Hillsdale) (GDN)
Betty Sue Sweeney, RN (Southwestern) (HD)
Jeanne Wineland, RN (Montcalm-Ionia) (GDN)
Ann Jones, RN (Grand Rapids) (PHN)
Isabelle Wallen, RN (Barry-Calhoun) (GDN)
Ruth Henkelmann, RN (Detroit) (EACT)
Connie Meade, RN (Capital Area) (PHN)
Diane Sobocienski, RN (Oakland) (PDN)

Avis Dykstra, RN, who served as MNA Associate Executive Secretary and was instrumental in developing MNA's Economic Security Program, wrote:

"MNA recommends that the base salary for the general duty nurse should be $400-500/month. This is exclusive of any fringe benefits…MNA should first and foremost concentrate intensive efforts on improved salaries so that nursing will compare favorably and appropriately with other occupations and professions. After salary adjustments, high priority will be given for improving fringe benefits, which will include retirement programs, life insurance, and hospital-medical insurance coverage for all nurses."

As the E&GW program developed, nursing practice continued to evolve. MNA issued a 1970 position paper on "Comprehensive Health Care" stating:

"Four basic conditions emerge which must be satisfied if the health needs of people – all people – are to be met and our human resources cherished and developed. The four conditions are availability, accessibility, acceptability, and accountability of health service systems to consumers for the nature, quantity and quality of health care provided though the systems."

Part of the comprehensive health discussion was the growing field of mental health. Public Act 54, passed by the Michigan Legislature in 1963 and amended in March 1966, provided that cities of 50,000 or more, or any county or combination of counties may establish or participate in a comprehensive mental health program. In 1971, MNA's Division of Psychiatric & Mental Health Nursing was very active and formed two division groups, the Advocates for Child Psychiatric Nursing and the Council for State-Employed Nurses.

Continuing education expanded, and in 1968 about 4,000 RNs attended conferences and workshops planned and sponsored by MNA. "Wednesday with MNA" was expanded to 13 spring conferences in 1969. Miss Patricia Camp, RN coordinated a series of continuing education workshops in 1970. Mrs. Harriett Sattig, RN was appointed as MNA Project Director for "Continuing Education of Nursing

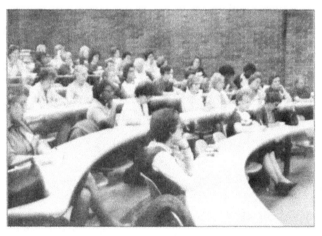

MNA members take the opportunity to broaden their professional experience by attending a "Wednesday with MNA" conference at the Art, Sciences and Career Building, Lansing Community College, Lansing.

Personnel in Michigan," funded in 1971 by a US Public Health Service Grant to survey the needs and resources for continuing education for licensed in nurses in Michigan.

In 1971, more than 300 registered nurses throughout Michigan were involved in study groups to assist the MNA Task Force on Nursing Practice in the development of an MNA Position Paper on Nursing Practice.

A program for nursing administrators, "Changing Needs and Changing Systems," was offered that year. To meet the growing need for continuing education, Elizabeth Peckham, RN joined the MNA staff in 1973 as the first Director for Nursing Practice.

The annual Nurses Week celebration, which moved from week to week until the mid-90s, provided MNA members an opportunity to explain the practice of nursing to the general public. The May 1969 issue of *The Michigan Nurse* reports "Two MNA members appeared on 'Formula,' a television program about professional organizations, broadcast over WJIM-TV, May 4, which opened a week-long observance of Michigan Nurse Week."

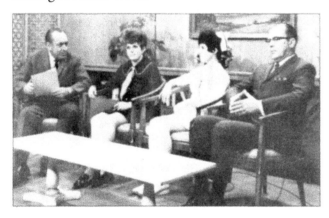

Molly Gee, RN, psychiatric nursing unit, St. Lawrence Hospital, Lansing (2nd from l) and Brigid Warren, RN, instructor and nurse clinician, School of Nursing, Michigan State University (3rd from l) joined Hugh W. Brenneman (l), host of "Formula" and Roger B. Nelson, MD (r) senior associate director, University Hospital, Ann Arbor in a discussion about nurses and their role on the health team.

Bay District RNs and LPNs combined to challenge the MDs to a basketball game as one of several activities used to observe Michigan Nurse Week, 1970. Other

activities observed included: attendance at church services in full uniform, an essay contest written by 6th graders on "Why I Would Like to Become a Nurse," and displays about nursing in local banks and at Delta College.

An increased opportunity for nursing education was celebrated during this time with the University of Michigan announcing a Nursing PhD and a baccalaureate program for "making provisions for previous achievement and current competencies" for registered nurses who graduated from an associates degree or diploma program.

"Shortage of New RNs Tied to Low Salaries," announced a headline in the first *ESP-Line,* a new insert in *The Michigan Nurse* beginning in July of 1967. There was again a shortage of nurses – which greatly impacted nursing practice and the pursuit of economic security. A headline in the March 1966 issue of *Good Housekeeping* stated, "If the blunt truth be known, patients in hospitals are getting less and less attention." In 1967, *The Michigan Nurse* reported a shortage of 5,000 RNs in the state.

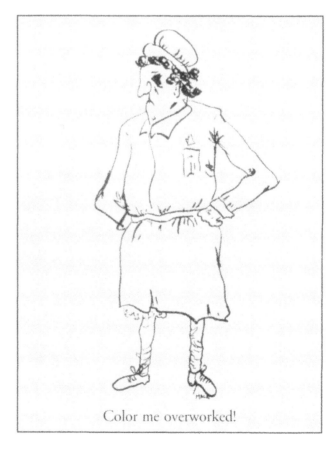

Color me overworked!

A survey of the over 15,000 inactive RNs conducted that year revealed three primary reasons why the RNs were not in the workforce: family responsibilities at home (47%), inability to work hours required of a nurse (14.6%), and nursing salaries not commensurate with expenses incurred by working (11%)."

Inactive RNs also indicated that they needed to be updated in order to return to practice. In response, MNA pioneered federal "RN Refresher Courses" for inactive registered nurses. These 240-hour refresher courses updated them in nursing theory and practice, thus enabling them to continue their professional careers. In 1967, MNA administered the first one-year $171,000 program for the Michigan Employment Security Commission, offering 22 programs, enrolling 408 RNs from 37 counties. The courses were a great success, and the contract was renewed annually through 1972.

MNA activities through the sixties and early seventies reflected the changing social climate as the 1968 HOD resolution resolved:

> "that the Michigan Nurses Association promote, practice and support principles and programs of good human relations within the nursing

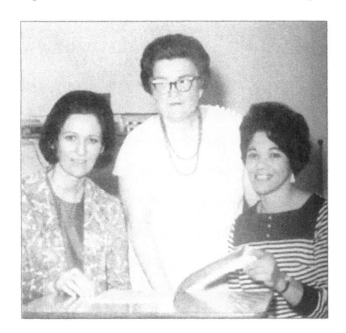

MNA's refresher course coordinator Ruth E. Blakeley, RN, (center) confers with instructors Genevieve A. Czarnecki, RN, (left) and Estelle Turner, RN (right).

profession which foster a climate conducive to the comfortable participation of ALL nurses in our profession and in the society."

Inroads into the profession for black nurses continued to be slow. Gladys Manzo, RN and Sarah Vaughn, RN, founded Detroit's Lambda Chi Chapter of the National Sorority, Chi Eta Phi, in 1965. Bernice F. Morton, PhD, RN, an Associate Professor in Nursing at Wayne State University, was the first African American to be appointed Department Chair in the College of Nursing and the first Minority Affairs Director for Nursing in 1968, and Geraldine H. Doby, RN, founded the Detroit Black Nurses' Association as one of thirteen chapters of the National Black Nurses Association.

The 1969 Annual Convention included a forum on "Issues of working women: How do they influence the professional and social role of the nurse?" The cost for convention was $2.50 for members; $5 for non-members. The 1969 HOD "adopted the proposed 1970 Legislative Program with the exception of support for liberalizing current Michigan abortion laws." And, in 1973, reflecting the growing concern for the environment, a HOD resolution noted that RNs "should become more actively involved in making themselves aware of problems in environmental quality."

And, while the nursing profession and educational system was having growing pains, so was the association. MNA was housed at 508 Hollister Building in Lansing, and had purchased a lot on Chester Road in Lansing Township. However, as Mrs. Elizabeth Vigeant, RN, chairman of the building committee reported in the January/February issue of *The Michigan Nurse*:

> "Then the East Lansing Trinity Church building became available. This is at 120 Spartan Avenue, just off Grand River, east of the MSU campus. This is our 'Winchester Cathedral,' the objective of the 'Spartan Team' effort. It'll make a dandy office."

After several tentative dates, MNA moved into the new building and dedicated it on Saturday, May 10, 1669. To accomplish the goal, members bought bonds, contributed their S&H Green Stamps, coupon cards, money, furniture and decorations, and raised $26,000 through a raffle at the 1968 convention.

In 1967, MNA had seven employees and 9,741 members, including new graduates (who joined MNA within six months of licensure) and "associates". By mid-year of 1969 the membership was at 7,066; flexible membership was implemented this year so an RN could join anytime in the year and get a full year of benefits.

In September 1971, Mrs. Joan S. Guy, RN, Executive Director wrote:

"If one measures program accomplishments as a kind of barometer for the health of the Association, we might forecast:

Membership – cloudy; holding somewhat steady

Legislation – fair; possible gusts and showers

Professional Nursing Practice – sunny and fair with brisk winds

Economic Security – partly cloudy, barometer holding steady; fair skies ahead

Continuing Education – clearing and blue skies

Communications – low cloud cover, gradual clearing

Liaison with Other Groups – generally fair; possible frost in low lying areas."

In the 70s, some of MNA administrative costs were offset by successful member travel plans, such as the Rhine cruise in 1972 and the Austrian Alpine adventure in 1973.

The Michigan Nurse became a quarterly magazine in 1970 with clinical and educational articles and other pertinent information. A quarterly newsletter, *ESP-Line,* containing news about legislation, district

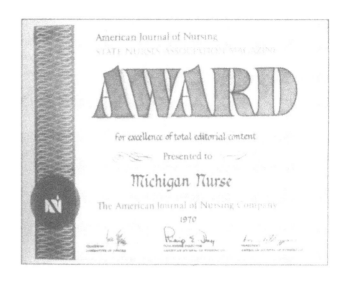

activities and other general features, was distributed at six-week intervals between issues of the magazine. With this arrangement, MNA won the *AJN* State Nurses' Association Magazine "Award for excellence of total editorial content".

"Accepting the awards at a luncheon honoring the SNAs were John H. Wick, RN, president (1967-71), MNA and Mrs. Joan S. Guy, RN, executive director, MNA. Awards were presented by Pat Walsh, RN, (Washtenaw) chairman of the *AJN* State Nurses Association awards committee."

First steps were taken in 1973 to develop and implement a CE Recognition Program, based on an earlier MNA-published continuing education study. Dorothy H. Coye, RN, chairperson of the Committee of Continuing Education, led the effort to pilot a CERP in seven districts in 1974 and 1975.

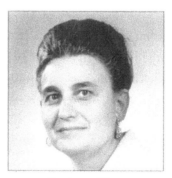

Barbara Horn

As this decade came to a close, Barbara J. Horn, RN, PhD (Washtenaw), a research associate at University of Michigan and chairperson of Task force on Nursing Practice, was elected president at MNA's 64th Annual convention in Grand Rapids.

Those Who Marched
Joan S. Guy, RN

by Jess Merrill

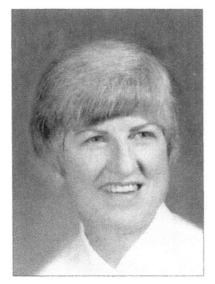

World War II was winding down when Joan S. Guy was beginning to consider career choices. Her decision to become a nurse was a combination of her orientation toward a service related profession, and the federal Cadet Nurse Corps, which funded education for nurses. By the time she had finished the diploma program, the Cadet Nurse program had been cancelled, and along with it both the obligation and the opportunity to serve as a military nurse.

Joan received her diploma in 1948 at the Presbyterian Hospital School of Nursing, Chicago, Illinois. Between graduation and 1956, Joan held various staff and head nurse positions in Illinois and Wisconsin. She completed her baccalaureate degree in psychology at Carroll College, Waukesha, Wisconsin in 1952, and did graduate work at Michigan State University after moving to Lansing, Michigan in 1956.

Joan and her husband moved to Michigan after he had been discharged from the Navy and accepted a position with Michigan Bell in Lansing, and Joan worked as a medical/surgical nurse at Sparrow Hospital.

She joined the staff of the Michigan Nurses Association in 1962 as Assistant Executive Director, and counselor, and then in 1968 she accepted the position of Executive Director, which she held until 1979 when she stepped down to become Associate Executive Director.

Her decision to give up the Executive Director position was fueled by the expansion and growth of programs in the Association, and she felt the organization needed someone better prepared in finance and general administration. She had also become deeply involved in the CURN program and wanted to guide that project to completion, which she did.

Among the pressing issues of the time were collective bargaining and the philosophical differences nurses held regarding the concept of unions and the appropriateness of the professional association to organize nurses for such purposes. Other issues were the slowness of the profession to upgrade and accept educational standards for nurses, and finding better ways to incorporate nursing research into clinical practice.

Joan is happily retired and living with her husband in Haslett, Michigan.

When asked if she would choose nursing as a career today, she said she would because there has rarely been a glut of nurses available, and, she added "... but I think I would take a different educational route. There are so many facets of nursing now that weren't available when I began."

Alpena General Hospital Staff Council

by Linda Canfield, RN

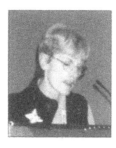

Alpena General Hospital (AGH) RNs are currently found in three separate bargaining units represented by MNA: staff nurses, supervisory nurses and home care nurses. The earliest mention of RNs in the Alpena area is from the December 1939 minutes of the Alpena District Nurses Association (ADNA). Earlier that year, ADNA had heard about nursing on the front during World War I from a Red Cross nurse. At the December 1939 meeting, the RNs gathered for a Christmas party and brought gifts for the Indian children from Hubbard Lake, an area south of Alpena.

In January 1940, there were 31 RNs employed at Alpena General Hospital. On October 23, 1940, a meeting was held of the "Nurses Club" at AGH. Minutes of this meeting suggest the "Nurses Club" may have been an early predecessor of a collective bargaining unit. The group was determined to send delegates to Lansing to discover if the Michigan State Nurses Association would represent Alpena nurses in the "staff nurse section" at the upcoming Convention. In October, 1950, the District included 21 members and 16 RNs from the Alpena area.

The first contract negotiated by MNA for the RNs at AGH went into effect on July 1, 1972. The first posting for an RN under the contract is dated January 24, 1973 and was for a full time position on the midnight shift in the Mental Health unit at AGH. At that time, the RNs in the collective bargaining unit included staff nurses and shift supervisors. Nursing departments were run by Assistant Directors of Nurses who were not members of the bargaining units. In 1994, the hospital entered into negotiations to create a separate bargaining unit for Home Care Services RNs and for Nursing Supervisory personnel, leading to the current structure of three groups of RNs represented by the Michigan Nurses Association. Alpena General Hospital currently has 216 RNs represented by MNA.

The collective bargaining units at AGH have a long tradition of supporting nursing students. Minutes from a September, 1948 meeting propose giving a scholarship of $300.00 to a student nurse which would cover three years of room, board, tuition, books and uniforms. On April 5, 1954, the Alpena General "Nurses Club" donated $100.00 to the Mt. Carmel School of Nursing for a nursing student scholarship. Today, the Staff Council RNs at AGH still donate funds for nursing students to attend the MNA and Michigan Nursing Students Association (MNSA) Annual Conventions.

Borgess Nurse Staff Council

By Becky Baldwin, RN

The Borgess Staff Nurses Council had its beginnings in 1972 in what was then known as Borgess Hospital. Unfair labor practices and inequalities drove the nurses to seek collective action to address the problems, which included starting wages for new nurses that were higher than those of nurses with seniority at the hospital and favoritism in awarding job transfers.

Organizing began, and 51% of the nurses signed cards requesting an election for representation. Although the name of another union also appeared on the ballot, Borgess nurses selected the Michigan Nurses Association to represent them in collective bargaining. They felt that MNA would not only secure their rights but would also enable them to grow professionally. The first contract was negotiated and signed, and all nurses were members of the bargaining unit by 1973.

Early Staff Council chairpersons provided guidance for the fledgling council, encouraging bargaining unit members to stand up for their rights and to work together for the profession. Several also served the profession on MNA committees. In a reverse twist, the MNA field representative for Borgess, for a time, was a former Borgess nurse.

In 1980, the contract expired, and an impasse with the hospital led to a 6-week strike. Nurses won the strike, demonstrating that they would stand together for the professional rights they deserved.

A unique benefit of one contract was swing pay. Nurses negotiated time-and-a-half pay for any nurse asked to work a swing shift and then return to their own shift within 72 hours. The pay applied to the first swing shift and the first normal shift.

Current contract benefits include a double time hourly wage for any mandated overtime if more than one hour, limits on floating requirements and reinforcements for regular employee schedules and protection against unilateral schedule changes. The contract establishes a cap of 60 hours per week, including regulary scheduled shifts and additional hours.

The most challenging part of being a bargaining unit is helping the staff nurses realize that THEY are the bargaining unit – not the Michigan Nurses Association. To educate the nurses that they are the union, more membership meetings are being held, a newsletter is sent in alternate months when there is no meeting, and a web page is up and running (www.bmcmnarn.com). Current officers are working hard to increase communication to the membership.

And the future of the Borgess Staff Nurse Council in the next century? It will depend on unit nurses becoming actively involved the staff council – an area of nursing that is not currently addressed much during their educational process. The current officers are committed to standing up for the rights of nurses and improving nursing at Borgess. They want to make Borgess the best place for nurses, and with the help of the Michigan Nurses Association, they just may reach that goal!

Congratulations to the Michigan Nurses Association for being around for one hundred years! We hope you are here for many more years to stand up for the rights of nurses and to advance the profession.

Current officers
Chairperson: Patricia Meave, RN
Vice Chairperson: Becky Baldwin, RN, CPAN
Secretary: Carolyn Vestal, RN
Treasurer: Lori Van Zoeren, RN
Grievance Representative: Janet Bestervelt, RN

Recipients of MNA E&GW Achievement Awards
Pat Berger, Cheryl McKee, Judi Mills, Cheryl West-Hopkins

Monroe County Health Department Staff Council

By Deb Zimmerman, RN and Connie Harvell, RN

In the early 1970s, employees of the Monroe County Health Department were seeking to organize with the Teamsters union. However, the nurses felt that if they were going to have representation, they wished to belong to a professional organization. They sought out the Mchigan Nurses Association for their representation, and the first contract was signed on July 13, 1971.

The first negotiation committee consisted of Chairperson Roberta Heiden, RN, Estelle Barrow, RN, and Darlene Wahr, RN. The first Monroe County Health Department unit organized with MNA consisted of approximately seven members.

In the 1990s, we had as many as 31 members. Our most recent contract was signed January 1, 2000, with 24 nurses in Unit I.

In 1998, the supervisors became more active in hiring and discipline. Labor laws prohibited them from being in the same union with the nurses they supervised. Unit II was formed for the supervisors in 1998. The unit has three members.

A significant point of earlier contracts was the "me too clause" which provided that if one bargaining unit in the county received a benefit, such as additional sick time or personal time, then all units automatically received it. Today, each benefit or change must be negotiated individually.

Ottawa County Health Department Staff Council

By Bev Plagenhof, RN

The earliest documents found for the Ottawa County Health Department Staff Council are a contract for 1968-69 and a charter member list dated September 21, 1972. Retired member Joann Lemmen, RN, remembers that the first negotiations were conducted directly with the Health Department's commissioners. She remembers being told that nurses were a dime a dozen and that anyone off the street could do their job. She remembers being told that because nurses were women and not supporting families, they should not expect to be paid as much as men.

The 1968 contract for a public health nurse indicated a starting salary of $7,220 dollars per year (or $3.47 per hour) plus 10¢ per mile for travel. A nurse was entitled to a maternity leave without pay as soon as her pregnancy was confirmed but required permission from her doctor to work past her seventh month of pregnancy.

Conditions began to improve in 1972 as the Michigan Nurses Association began negotiating for the nurses. A staff council of 10 grew to 45 members. Nonetheless, bargaining has been very difficult, and significant gains would have been impossible without the help of MNA. Gains and issues included:

1981 – The County wanted to change the work day from 8:30-5 to 8-5 without an increase in pay. The nurses won this battle, but it was difficult.

1988 – A male nurse was hired at a higher wage than was posted because a doctor threatened to quit if the man were not paid more. After filing sex discrimination and unequal pay charges with MDCR and a unit clarification request with MERC, the issue was resolved. It took two years.

1968 - 2001 – Uniform issues were a problem for over 30 years. From a standard uniform, the nurses progressed to a dress code. What constituted a violation of the dress code became an issue. An initially non-existent uniform allowance changed to an allowance of $100 in 1971. Later, the allowance was threatened. Ultimately, in 2001, nurses exchanged the uniform allowance for a reduction in their pension cost. Today, nurses can wear professional attire of their choosing.

1992 – Fact finding, led by John Karebian of MNA and bolstered by the support of involved nurses, led to a successful contract which included part time benefits for nurses working a minimum of 16 hours per week. To date, this is the only bargaining unit with that benefit.

2001 – After the nurses approved a tentative agreement, the Board of Commissioners refused to approve it. Four months later, after intensive work by unit members and filing an Unfair Labor Practice charge, the contract was signed.

2004 – Ending over a year of negotiations and working without a contract, nurses ratified a new contract on April 6. The wage package is at least a 7.5 increase over the next three years of the contract, including retroactive pay for 2003. Sick leave and bereavement benefits were increased, as was the amount nurses are allocated for an annual physical. The types of immunizations that the county will administer to nurses without charge was expanded. In a hard-fought victory, nurses were also successful in limiting the percentage of health insurance cost increase they would be responsible to cover.

Yes, we have come a long way, but with challenges ahead, we need the one strong voice of MNA.

Visiting Nurse Services of Western Michigan Staff Council

by Bette O'Connor-Rogers, RN

Visiting Nurse Services was originally established and housed in the Kent County Public Health Department (KCHD) and went by the name of Community Health Service (CHS). Over time the name was changed to VNS of Western Michigan (VNS) after joining the nationwide Visiting Nurses Association (VNA). It was unusual in that, while a totally separate business, it was run and managed by the KCHD. Though working in the same environment, in the same building with desks side by side, CHS nurses were separate from the KCHD nursing staff and worked exclusively for CHS.

In the late 1960s, the KCHD nurses unionized. For a few years the two groups of nurses continued to work side by side. The CHS nurses remained non-unionized though they did benefit from the negotiations done by the nurses in the health department. After awhile it felt somewhat awkward not to be unionized too. So, wishing to join their professional union, the CHS nurses sought out the MNA, and in early 1969, the RN Staff Council of CHS was established. This first group started with four to five nurses and has grown to as much as 75 nurses at one time and now, with the onset of PPS (Perspective Payment System established by the Federal Government), it is at its current number of 62 nurses. At the first negotiation there was no legal representative for either side. The nurses and VNA Board representatives sat down together to collaboratively work out their first contract and then sent it to legal representation to get it written up "properly".

Today, the issues for which the union works are very different from when the union was established. The nurses continue to work for improved staffing and benefits including health care. They struggle with workload issues/mandatory overtime and continue to work to have a meaningful voice in their work environment. Working with the Visiting Nurse Services management has traditionally been a positive collaborative effort and has not been characterized by negativity and adversarial behavior. The Staff Council believes this has helped a great deal to continue the prosperity that the VNS has enjoyed over many years and has helped to maintain quality staff to provide quality care for our patients, their families and the community.

1974-1983

by Carol Feuss

Technology Explodes, Social Issues Impact MNA, and its Structure Evolves

Rapid technological change was the rule of this decade, as pocket calculators made slide rules obsolete, the IBM PC was designed, and in 1984 the Apple Macintosh introduced a "mouse" as part of their Personal Computer (PC). Space exploration was at its peak as the Viking mission went to Mars, Voyager was sent to explore the outer solar system, and the Space Shuttle *Challenger* had ten successful missions. A second shuttle, *Discovery*, was launched.

And change was not limited to technology. In 1975, the fear of nuclear war was dominant; there was high inflation and high unemployment; and OPEC oil was embargoed. It was the International Women's Year. Michigan had ratified the Equal Rights Amendment (ERA), but it had failed to pass nationally. As the decade progressed, the call for women's liberation, greater equality, and greater environmental awareness grew. Pop culture mourned the death of "the king," Elvis Presley, and celebrated the release of Pac-Man and *Star Wars*. In 1981, violence again visited an American President as Ronald Reagan was shot but not killed.

The increasing speed of developing technology and system changes impacted healthcare during this time as well. In 1980, smallpox was declared eradicated. As this decade in MNA's history opened, an amendment to the National Labor Relations Act was going into effect. This law repealed the prior exemption of the health care industry from coverage by the federal statues regulating labor relations and established a procedure for elections and collective bargaining in non-profit and voluntary hospitals.

The MNA House of Delegates resolutions reveal how society's issues had penetrated the organization over the decade. The House supported:

- the prohibition of using Medicare reimbursement for anti-union activities;

- a bilateral, variable nuclear freeze between the US and the USSR;
- limits on the amount of Poly Brominated Biphenyl Contamination (PBB);
- ANA's decision to only hold conferences in ERA ratified states;
- the international boycott of Nestle products because of the company's "misrepresentation of nursing to promote its product" and its "unethical and deceptive promotion tactics of infant formulas;"
- a *Newsweek* boycott over the October 1982 article, "Our Undertrained Nurses;"
- boycotting convention centers which demonstrate anti-labor policies; and
- sanctions against temporary agencies that cross picket lines.

Ann Zuzich was elected as president (1975-79) at the 1975 convention; Dorothea Milbrandt (1979-1983) and Regina Williams (1983-1985) provided presidential leadership the rest of the decade. During this time, Joan S. Guy served as Executive Director until 1979 when she stepped down to focus on membership development. Nadine M. Furlong was Executive Director until Carol Franck assumed the position in 1986.

"What is nursing practice? Who defines it? And what is nursing's scope of practice? These questions dominated the decade as reflected by the title of the 1975 convention: "Who Controls Nursing Practice?" held at the Olds Plaza Hotel in Lansing.

The Public Health Statute Revision Project (PHSRP) was established in 1975 to "streamline and standardize licensing laws covering individual health providers." MNA members worked with the Michigan Licensed Practical Nurse Association, the Licensed Psychiatric Nurses, and the Michigan Association of Nurse Anesthetists to develop a new definition of nursing practice based upon on the concept of a "scope of practice." *The Michigan Nurse* reported, "Monitoring proposals for a revised state public health code became

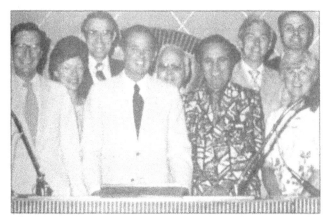

Governor William Milliken signs the new Health Code, while a group of consumers and providers look on including Joan S. Guy, RN, MNA Executive Director (right front).

MNA's top priority for 1976." After several years of work groups, drafts and public hearings, the new public health code (Public Act 368 of 1978), which included a recodification of all Michigan public health laws, went into effect on September 30, 1978. The new code also expanded the Board of Nursing's role to include setting standards and criteria for specialty certification of nurse midwives, nurse anesthetists and nurse practitioners. Under the new Code, there was a thirteen-member Board of Nursing with three registered nurses, two practical nurses and two public members.

ANA certification for nurse practitioners became a reality in 1975 when Martha M. Tousley, RN, a psychiatric nurse practitioner from Traverse City, was the first nurse in Michigan to receive ANA certification.

After several years of discussion and proposals, legislation defining physician assistants (PA) was passed in early 1977. Public Act 420 specified that PAs could prescribe drugs as a delegated act. An Attorney General opinion later that year clarified that "physician assistants are legally dependent in their practice to licensed approved physicians whereas nurses function under an independent license and are directly accountable to the recipient of care."

President Jimmy Carter signed the Rural Health Clinic Services legislation in December of 1977 which required the Medicare and Medicaid programs to pay for the service of nurse practitioners and physician assistants in rural, medically underserved areas.

MNA members voiced a growing concern about temporary nursing personnel in health agencies, especially long term care facilities. The MNA Division of Administration was directed by the 1974 House of Delegates to develop guidelines for the use of supplemental nursing services. The guidelines were then sent to the director of the Office of Long Term Care at the US Public Health Service (HEW) with the question, "Do the federal rules and regulations allow temporary personnel to be counted in staffing requirements?" Chief Nurse Officer and Assistant Surgeon General Fay G. Abdellah, PhD answered in part, "…the hazards of using temporary personnel have been correctly identified, and facilities should be made aware that such a practice does run the risk of non-certification…" MNA continued to watch the trend with concern and updated its "Use of Supplemental Nursing Services" guidelines in 1981.

MNA was part of the Nursing Home Reform Coalition, which saw the successful passage in September of 1979 of SB 659, sponsored by Senator John Otterbacher. The bill mandated that nursing homes "retain 2.25 hours nursing care per patient, per day." It further specified that directors of nursing must be an RN with a background in gerontology and that a licensed nurse (LPN or RN) must be on duty 24 hours/day.

MNA was involved in the State Health Plan Committee, which was required as part of the amended National Health Planning and Resources Development Act of '74 and PA 323 of 1978. Barbara Chadwick chaired MNA's involvement in the early '80s. MNA submitted recommendations in all areas: health services, health facilities, health personnel and cost. Specific recommendations were made regarding the size and preparation of the nurse work force as predicted for 1983-87.

The ongoing discussion about scope of practice and the role of nursing in the health care system drove the need for additional research. The August 1975 issue of *The Michigan Nurse* announced:

"MNA received a five-year grant by the Division of Nursing, US Department of Health, Education and Welfare, to increase the use of findings from nursing research in daily practice, to support modifications in research findings that will help nurses use new knowledge on the job and to provide financial support for research directly related to nursing practice in selected hospitals in the state."

The CURN Project, (Conduct and Utilization of Research in Nursing), began under the direction of Maxine Loomis. JoAnne Horsley, RN, PhD, Chairperson for the Council on Nursing Research in 1975, became the principle investigator as the project progressed. Based on preliminary data collected in 18 hospitals and from a survey of 800 RNs, a handbook was developed by CURN staff to assist nurses in conducting trials and evaluating the results of a nursing innovation. Ten protocols on "Using Research to Improve Nursing Practice" were also developed, and sold from $8.50 to $14.50 each.

The MNA board decided that "if materials from the CURN Project are published, that MNA royalties be kept in separate funds for the purpose of supporting the major goals of the project." As a result, the CURN Competitive Research Award program was created. Christine Gmeiner, RN, MS, was granted the first MNA CURN Competitive Research Award Grant

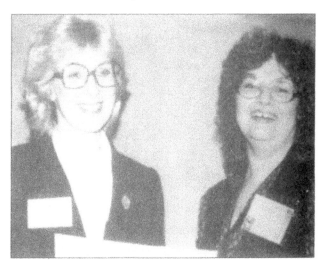

The first CURN scholar, Christine Gmeiner, RN, CS, (l) is presented with a check by Dr. Marjorie Isenberg.

based on her research in "Patient Behavior Care Needs, Family and Community Resources of Both Institutionalized and Non-Institutionalized Alzheimer's Patients."

There were also legal issues impacting both the MNA structure and nursing practice as national and local organizations struggled with the implications of the new changes to the Labor-Management Relations Act (Taft-Hartley Act). In a 1974 amendment, the National Labor Relation Board (NLRB) rules now covered proprietary hospitals and health care institutions. Although Michigan nurses had the right to bargain collectively for some years, the amendment meant that registered nurses would no longer be included with any non-professionals unless they voted for such an inclusion. The Division of Administration Executive Committee Chair, Margaret Morrow, RN, noted in 1975:

> "This is a time of upheaval and unrest in the definition of the role of the nurse in this particular aspect of practice (nursing administration). It is hoped some legal decisions will help settle questions regarding the relationship of nursing administrators to the professional nursing organization."

This discussion and struggle has continued through the years.

In the meantime, membership was growing through the chartering of new staff councils. In 1975, E&GW Council Chairperson Arlouine Fende reported that six charters were issued to staff councils, and 58 contracts were negotiated or in the process of being negotiated. Among the charters was the University of Michigan Hospital, which became the state's largest local bargaining council of nurses, with 800 in the unit. In 1976 it was reported that over 50% of MNA members were in staff councils.

A Continuing Education Labor Program was initiated by the E&GW Commission in 1978 to strengthen the new staff councils. In addition to leadership workshops, conferences on specific topics such as nursing power and the law, verbal skills in negotiations,

grievance procedures, contract enforcement, and assertiveness training were offered.

Members of the 1978 commission included: Karen Schrader, Becky Sue Baldwin, Madonna Balance, Margo Barron, Larry Bontrager, Marilyn Glidden, Nancy Sullivan, and Bruce Tucker.

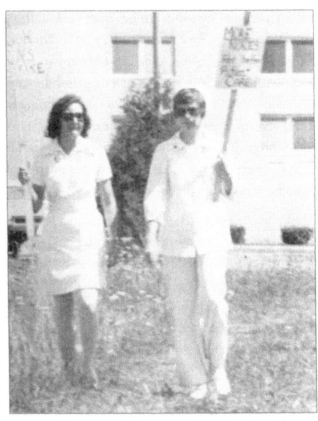

Registered nurses picketing outside Lansing General Hospital.

E&GW staff members were busy as local leadership struggled to make nursing practice and economic gains. In addition to the many successful contract negotiations, work stoppages marked this decade as well. Lansing General Hospital nurses went on a three-week strike in 1977 as they struggled to gain respect and have a nursing practice committee recognized.

The 1978 Riverside Osteopathic Hospital strike centered around the "hospital's refusal to offer the nurses health care benefits other area nurses currently receive." The nurses were quoted in the *Michigan Nurse* as saying:

"When an expensive piece of life-saving machinery arrives at a hospital, no one complains about the costs. But when the people who provide direct patient care ask for equal benefits and salaries comparable with other workers, they are blamed for the rising cost of health care."

Wayne County Professional Nurse Council, representing 435 RNs from seven county facilities, was ordered back to work 17 hours after withdrawing their services in early December, 1978. Their work stoppage was to emphasize the need for improved patient-care standards and professional working conditions.

Baraga County (L'Anse) Memorial Hospital Staff RNs' 1978 contract included leaves of absence for Association business, tuition reimbursement, professional nursing practice and patient care special conferences, and inclusion of the ANA/MNA "Role of the Nurse" language in the agreement.

In a situation unique to this decade, Wayne County Professional Nurse Council filed a grievance in 1976 which "said they believed the employer's requirement that female nurses wear caps constituted sex discrimination since there was no such requirement for male nurses." The labor board agreed and the nurses won the right to "choose not to wear caps." Borgess Hospital nurses went to arbitration in 1979 over a grievance affirming nursing's right to operate as a separate functioning component of hospital operation.

The Dickinson County Memorial Hospital Staff Council survived an attempt in 1984 to break up their unit, which consisted of staff nurses, head nurses and house supervisors. After nearly a year of negotiations by Carolyn Rose, Joyce Erickson, Mary Negro, Pat

Dennis, Nancy Theisen, Elizabeth Beal, and Linda Yoder, the nurses gained a new contract – after a strike vote was called. Carole Keiller, RN, MNA Field Representative, reported the nurses received an average wage increase of 12.2%, additional compensation for an air ambulance run, parent leave, and 100% tuition reimbursement.

Organizing new units was impacted by two decisions in the early '80s. The May 1982 *E&GW News*, written by Joan M. Goff, RN, and Jesse Bateau, RN, reported a change in membership policy:

> "MNA will now file an election petition with only 10% MNA membership and 60% authorization cards. Previously 51% membership in MNA was required before assistance was given in organization of a new unit."

One of the 1982 MNA HOD Resolutions stated:

> "Whereas: one of MNA's long range goals is to pursue representing all RNs in need of and eligible for collective bargaining...be it resolved: that MNA assign or employ an individual with appropriate skills and experience in organizing whose responsibilities will be to respond to inquiries and to seek and organize new staff councils."

The evolution of nursing education continued as the MNA Division of Education authored "Facts for RNs Returning to School" in 1975. Later that year, the first graduate program for family nurse clinicians was developed by the MSU School of Nursing with funding from the W.K. Kellogg Foundation. The first nursing PhD was awarded in 1978 at the University of Michigan to Marcia DeCann Anderson.

	Practical Nursing	Hospital Diploma	Associate Degree	Baccalaureate Degree	Masters Degree	Total RN
Educational Programs in Nursing, 1964-1974						
1964	23	22	5	5	2	32
1974	38	14	19	10	2	43
%	65% increase	36% decrease	280 increase	100% increase	-	34%*
						*(% change 64-74)

History of the University of Michigan Professional Nurse Council

By John Armelagos, RN, BSN and Jody Berney, RN

In 1974, RNs employed at the University of Michigan Medical Center desired to advance their professional aspirations and promote higher quality patient care through collective bargaining. On February 10, 1975, the employer recognized the University of Michigan Professional Nurse Council (UMPNC) with MNA as their exclusive representative.

On April 12, 1976, the first contract was forged which covered the approximate 800 staff nurses, health nurses, nursing education coordinators, Clinical Nurse Specialists, and Nurse Anesthetics. The contract was a mere 83 pages, but a tremendous achievement for UMPNC.

In 1978, UMPNC established their primary responsibility was patient care, and not non-nursing roles. This demand for recognition of RN professional autonomy and clinical authority continues to this day.

In 1989, UMPNC had grown to 1,800 members and bargained seven contracts with the University. The use of mandatory overtime for staffing and unrealistic shifts for senior nurses, which had been persistent problems for many years, led to a work stoppage when lines were drawn. After the settlement, both sides began to explore whether there could be another model that could meet their respective obligations without the combative approach of traditional bargaining.

After much negotiation, the two groups created the first contract under mutual gains bargaining. One of the successful outcomes is the joint creation of a shared governance model concerning clinical practice. With the 2001 contract

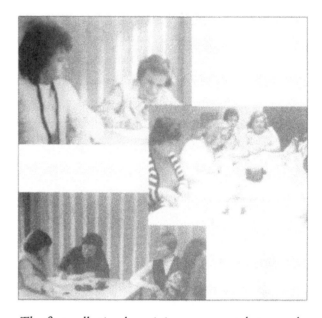

The first collective bargaining agreement between the University of Michigan and the Michigan Nurses Association is signed on April 12. Signing for the University (top l-r) are Becky Mason, RN, and Marge Jackson, RN, Director of Nursing. (Center) University of Michigan bargaining teams (from left): Vicki Neiberg, MNA Field Representative; Margo Barron, RN, Staff Council Chair; Phyllis Baldwin, RN, and Carolyn Gilbert, RN, Staff Council; (not pictured – Grace Oldenbroek, Bill Neff and Doug Geister, U of M Personnel Department, and Doug Ryckman, Administrator, Mott Hospital). (Bottom) MNA bargaining team members (from left) Leslie Pratt, RN, Ozella Wadley, RN, Beverly Pavasaris, RN, and Amy Goldberg, RN.

UMPNC finally gained tangible limits on mandatory overtime.

The 2004 UMPNC membership boasts more than 2,700 RNs with leaders across the state and nation, serving as MNA delegates, members of the MNA Board of Directors, MNA officers, MNA Economic and General Welfare Cabinet members, and delegates to UAN and ANA.

In 1977, MNA published a "Position Paper on Graduate Education in Nursing in Michigan," which identified a critical shortage of clinical nurse specialists, nurse faculty, nurse supervisors/administrators, and nurse researchers in light of intense student demand and numerous employment opportunities. It also recorded the transition in nursing education toward associate and baccalaureate degrees preparation.

Following a failure rate of 12.4% on the RN exams during 1973-77, the Board of Nursing discontinued issuing temporary permits in 1978, which had allowed new graduate nurses to practice before passing the state boards.

The issue of entry into practice has a long and convoluted history in the nursing profession. For many years at the American Nurses Association's House of Delegates, position papers were developed, debated and some adopted, calling for the BSN as the minimal educational level for licensure as a registered nurse. A number of deadlines were set and passed for legislation to be enacted in each state (1965, 1985, etc.).

MNA engaged in statewide forums beginning in 1979 in preparation for adopting the "1985 position." This position caused considerable controversy within the profession and within MNA.

In 1979, MNA's Entry into Practice Task Force recommended two categories of nursing practice: professional nursing practice with BSN minimum; and "the other category practice" with an ADN. They also recommended separate sets of competencies developed at the national level for these two levels of nursing.

The MNA was part of the Michigan Coalition on Articulation in Nursing Education (M-CANE) in 1980. M-CANE's goals were to make it easier for RNs to get a BSN, and for RNs to move from one school to another as part of the educational process.

In the early eighties, nursing and nursing education were crippled by federal budget cuts for nursing education. Funding for nursing education went from nearly $100 million in 1981; to $49 million in 1982;

to $12.5 million in 1983. The result created a crisis nationally, as the American Hospital Association estimated 100,000 budgeted vacancies for RNs in hospitals alone while colleges of nursing were closing their doors due to the funding cuts.

This crisis was brought home to Michigan as Michigan State University President Cecil Mackey recommended that the MSU College of Nursing be eliminated. The MSU President is quoted as saying, "…the Nursing Program is not essential for the college of medicine to achieve their primary objective."

MNA members joined with MSU students and alumni to fight the decision. MSU Trustee Peter Fletcher, R-Ypsilanti, was quoted in the *Detroit News* as saying, "I have never seen a better organized political effort…in my entire career."

Press conferences, testimony at the MSU board meetings, over 300 articles, editorials and letters in Michigan newspapers, and 6,000 letters to the chair of the MSU board were effective. On April 4, 1981, the MSU board voted to keep the College, but reduced the class size to 100.

In 1983 the National Council Licensing Examination (NCLEX) replaced the State Board Test Pool examination and CB-McGraw-Hill replaced the National League of Nursing as the testing agency.

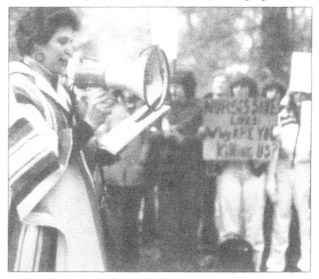

MNA Executive Director Nadine Furlong raises the spirits of MSU nursing students rallying to protest the proposed closing of the College of Nursing.

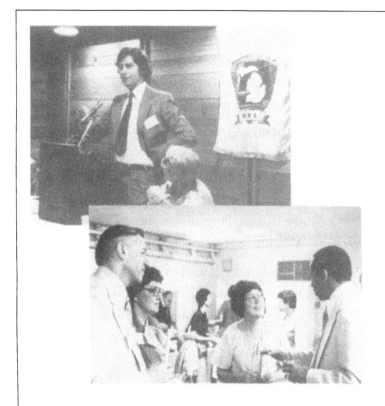

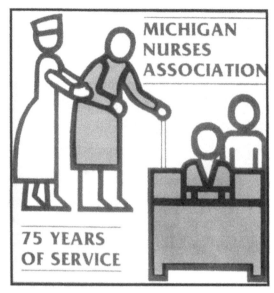

(Above top) During a series of programs and open houses, Harold H. Gardner, MD, Health Care Institute executive director, explains his controversial position on the RN-MD relationship and State Representative Joe Young (D-Detroit), (at right in lower photo) discusses legislative concerns with MNA members and staff. (Above right) Artwork from the July, 1979 cover of the "Michigan Nurse".

MNA celebrates its Diamond Jubilee

MNA celebrated its Diamond Jubilee on May 10-12, 1979. The convention theme was "2004: Can We Get There From Here?" The main session was "Nursing – an essential public service," with ANA President Barbara Nichols, RN, MASN; State Representative William A. Ryan; (D-Detroit); and *Detroit Free Press* medical writer Dolly Katz. Other program sessions included: "The Art and Politics of Decision Making," "The Nurse Practitioner – Distinguishing Between Nursing and Medical Practice," and "Nursing: 1904-2004."

The continuing education topics offered during this decade are revealing as new topics surfaced: ambulatory care, nurses as independent practitioners, cancer, and Sudden Infant Death. As this aspect of the association grew, funding was received from the Division of Nursing and the Department of Health, Education and Welfare (HEW) for a study on CE needs and resources for RNs in Michigan. The results of this study became the basis for MNA to seek accreditation from the American Nurses Association as a provider and approver of continuing education in nursing. MNA first achieved accreditation as a provider and approver in 1977.

For the approval function, Regional Review Boards were established geographically throughout the state. These boards accomplished significant educational endeavors, teaching nurses about ANA CE standards that must be used to plan and present their conferences and workshops.

More than 200 individual offerings were reviewed for approval in 1983-84, and an average of 14 CE programs provided by structural units were facilitated in each of those years. MNA also offered an accrual record system for RNs where their participation in approved programs was recorded in a central file system available upon request.

Always looking for new ways to make nurses and nursing more visible, 1978 was pronounced the national Year of the Nurse. MNA identified March as "Spend a Day with a Nurse" month. Each district was encouraged to invite a high profile community member to shadow a nurse. A sixty-second public service announcement, "Think About Nursing," which highlighted family-centered nursing at Family Hospital in Milwaukee was also produced.

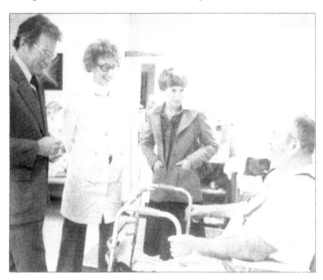

EMU president James Brickley spending "A Day with a Nurse" with Judie Wood, RN, Marilyn Welch, RN (Washtenaw-Monroe District), an instructor at EMU's Department of Nursing, and a client of the facility.

Although the idea of dividing the Legislation Committee into two separate branches had been discussed in 1973, MNA's first step toward a political action committee (PAC) was at the 1977 convention when INPUT (Involved Nursing Politically United Together) was formed. INPUT was:

> "a voluntary, unincorporated, non-profit organization for nurses and others interested in improving health care through the political process. It is politically non-partisan and operates collaboratively with other nursing organizations."

Annual dues were $10 and $3 for students. INPUT became the official PAC of MNA in 1984.

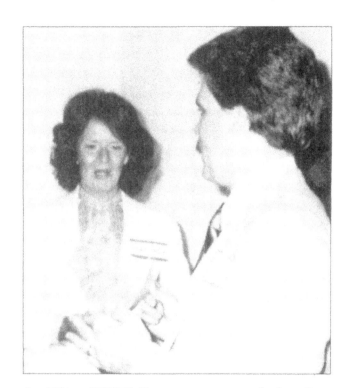

Joe White, INPUT Treasurer, presents a check to State Representative Debbie Stabenow, who was endorsed by INPUT in her 1984 re-election campaign.

At the national level, Michigan's influence remained strong. President Carter appointed MNA member Ellen Zimmerman to a National Advisory Committee of the White House Conference on Aging in 1980. The MNA Division of Gerontological Nursing Practice sponsored a Mini-White House conference Community Forum the next year. Merrie Jean Kaas, was the Chairperson and Janet Holloway was the Secretary.

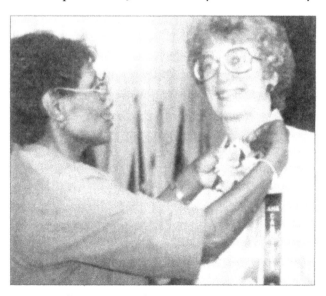

Regina Williams congratulates MNA member Sally Sample (right) on her election to the ANA Board of Directors.

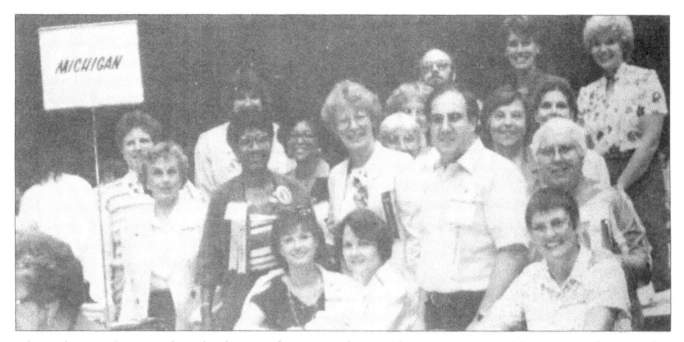

The Michigan Delegation takes a break to pose for a group photo. Michigan was represented by Regina Williams, Nadine Furlong, Gary Viele, Jesse Bateau, Rita Gallagher, Lilo Heolzel-Seipp, Sandy Spoelstra, Beverly Jones, Karen Brown, Rochelle Igrisan, Elizabeth Peckham, Pat Underwood, Joann Wilcox, Margo Barron, Phyllis Walker, Betty Bryant, Joanne Easterling, Debrah Hartwick, Marge Jackson, Kathy Cowley, Mary Neff, Sandy Wilson, Pat West, Reg Williams, and Lucy Brand.

In 1981, Phyllis M. Walker, RN, reported on her trip to Tokyo, Japan as an ANA volunteer at the ICN conference, "Health Care for All: Challenge for Nursing."

As the Equal Rights Amendment (ERA) struggled to pass, MNA members were deeply involved in discussing the "concept of comparable worth." In 1978, Chief Judge Fred Winner of the US 10th District Court ruled against registered nurses in *Lemmons vs. City of Denver*, saying the law "allows the comparison of male and female nurse salaries but does not require a comparison with salaries paid for non-health related jobs." In 1980 white women earned 63% and African American women earned 58% of the average white male weekly earnings. Growing frustration is reflected in a1982 HOD resolution that:

- "endorses the concept of comparable worth that recognized equal compensation for employees performing work of comparable worth or value regardless of their sex,"

- "urges the MNA BOD to take all measures deemed necessary for promoting and strengthening the growing movement for securing economic justice for women employees, including nurses, by supporting legislation, litigation and research aimed at strengthening the movement,"

- "registered nurses in their employment situation be encouraged to challenge reliance upon current rates of compensation as a validating factor in determining salary structures because current rates are themselves based on past economic discrimination."

E&GW Commission members represented MNA at the State of Michigan Comparable Worth Task Force meetings in 1984. MNA Executive Director Nadine M. Furlong, RN noted in one of several comparable worth articles in the *Michigan Nurse* that year:

"RNs have been underpaid since the inception of the profession…The wage and salary concerns of all women are embodied in the wage and salary concerns of nurses. No other female occupation provides such a glaring example of the failure of market forces to determine appropriate wage rate. If market forces responded to supply and demand, the severe shortages of registered nurse would lead to higher wages. Instead hospitals respond to shortages by substituting less skilled workers, attempting to lower standards of preparation and importing nurses from other countries rather than raise wages."

The MNA Commission on Human Rights, formalized in 1978, addressed other kinds of discrimination. Theressa Dixon, RN, served as the first chairperson; Doris Stewart, RN, David Hickman, RN, and Emily Cleveland, RN were the first members. The Commission was assigned to create "conscious raising" procedures with and for others in the membership to increase the involvement of minorities. The Commission authored a series of articles in 1981 and 1982:

"to call attention to the health needs of the disabled, disadvantaged, frail or high risk populations in our society for which nursing and nurses share accountability to serve and protect." A small victory was celebrated in 1983 when 500 nurses from nine nursing organizations held a welcome reception for Gloria Smith, PhD, RN, the new Director of the Michigan Department of Public Health. Dr. Smith was the first woman, first black woman, and first nurse to hold this position."

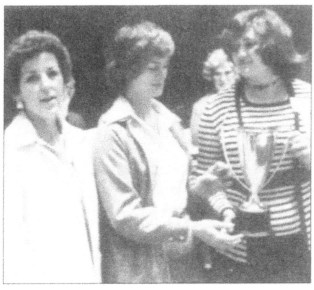

Lenawee District Delegates Dorothy Pennington, Kathy Rainone and Ann Itter accept the membership trophy for recruiting the greatest percentage of members in 1977.

With so many changes, the MNA Board and House of Delegates persevered in trying to find the right Association structure – in fact, this would be a major focus from 1979-84. The discussion of how to grow the membership resulted in a Membership/Marketing Committee which initiated, among other tactics, a district competition.

A snapshot of MNA members in 1980 revealed that MNA membership mirrored the Michigan nurse population except in the area of educational preparation, which showed more MNA members with a baccalaureate degree or higher:

Education Level	Diploma	Associate	Bac +
MNA Members	53.8%	19.8%	26.4%
All in MI	64.0	21.1	14.8

Employment Setting
Hospitals	70.0%
Community Health	13.0%
Nursing Homes	2.4%
Education	7.6%
Other	7.0%

Position
Staff Nurse	62.0%
Head Nurse	9.0%
Nursing Administrator	12.2%
Nurse Educators/Other	16.8%

Age
Under 29	28.0%
30-39	26.0%
40-49	18.3%
50-59	16.0%
60+	11.7%

Gender
Female	97.9%
Male	2.1%

Ethnicity
White	92.5%
Black	5.0%
Oriental	2.5%

In 1981, financial pressure was forcing changes in the organization. The Detroit district released staff, discontinued their registry service, and recommended that districts be combined. A survey of the Macomb district found that members preferred fewer meetings, and that regionalization might be a solution to dwindling involvement.

In 1982, the Board structure was changed to have 15, rather than 24 directors. This included the President, VP, Treasurer, Secretary, E&GW Commission, one representative each from the divisions of Administration, Community Health, Maternal/Child Health, Gerontology, Education Medical/Surgical, Psychiatric/Mental Health, three district representatives and one representative of New Graduates.

In September, 1984, as the MNA Finance Committee introduced a dues increase proposal, MNA had 6,810 members. (Michigan had 86,801 RNs at the time.) A $15 dues increase was approved which included funding for $45,000 of computer equipment to make dues collection faster and more accurate.

Twelve districts provided annual reports that year. Houghton district reported:

"Our group is experiencing great difficulty in attracting members to participate in local district activities. Administrative personnel in some facilities are discouraging participation by those nurses who are not covered by a staff council contract. Staff council members seldom participate in district functions. This causes a lack of cohesiveness in the local nursing community."

Kalamazoo reported an increased in membership by 101 members. Macomb counted 116 members, Northern Tri-County 114 members, Saginaw 126 members, and Washtenaw-Livingston-Monroe was the largest district by far, with 1,213 members.

As the decade closed, MNA employed a staff of 25 in the departments of Nursing Practice, Government Affairs, Education, Membership, Communications, E&GW and Administration. The cost of dues was about "$18 a month or 60 cents/day." The commissions became cabinets; councils became practice sections, and a study was underway to combine some of the 35 internal structural units to simplify the "cumbersome, excessively complex" organization.

1984-1993

by Carol Feuss

Communism Falls, AIDS is Prevalent, and the Internet Connects Humankind

Millions of Americans, including many school children, saw the Space Shuttle Challenger explode 74 seconds after lift-off in 1986, sending the space program into disarray.

The world community celebrated the fall of the Berlin Wall in 1989 and with it, much of communism. In the 1990s the Soviet Union ceased to exist, becoming the Commonwealth of Independent States, and American soldiers (including 200 Michigan nurses) were involved in Operation Desert Shield and Operation Desert Storm.

Life in America was transformed with the introduction of the Internet. The personal computer and the Internet connected people to information, people, and events around the world. In 1993, one in three Americans worked part of the time from home. Three out of four US homes owned VCRs, which became the fastest selling domestic appliance in history.

New acronyms such as AIDS (Acquired Immune Deficiency Syndrome), DRGs (Diagnosis-Related Group system), ADA (Americans with Disabilities Act of 1990), and FMLA (The Family and Medical Leave Act of 1993) became familiar terms in the health care setting. There was an over-supply of physicians, and RN positions were reduced as hospital censuses dropped; competition between physicians and nurses in primary care increased. And a massive reform of health care was proposed.

In September of 1985, Theressa Dixon, RN, chairperson of the Michigan Board of Nursing, reported that in Michigan there were 13 baccalaureate degree, 33 associate degree, 5 diploma (two of which had identified closing dates) and 29 practical nurse programs approved by the Board.

As Regina Williams, MNA's first African-American President finished her term in 1985, membership was at 6,915 and on the rise, with seventeen districts increasing their membership. Top percentage increases in a six month period: Newaygo (45%); Jackson (22%), Midland (14%) Barry-Calhoun (12%) and Lapeer (7%).

MNA moved ahead with Joann Wilcox as President from1985-1989, Patricia Underwood from1989 through 1993, and Linda Mondoux from1993 through 1997. MNA Director of Government Affairs Carol Franck assumed the Executive Director position in 1986.

After extensive and prolonged discussion and study, a major restructuring was implemented in 1986. Bylaws were changed to reflect the new structure and to further insulate the E&GW program from MNA Board of Directors influence.

Cabinets – Economic and General Welfare; Administration & Education; Nursing Research; and Nursing Practice, (with five practice sections: Community Health, Gerontology, Maternal/Child Health, Medical-Surgical, and Psych/Mental Health); Committees – Professional Affairs (Human Rights and Legislation) and Internal Affairs (Bylaws, CEARP, CE Advisory, Convention Program, Finance, Impartial, Nominations, Membership/Marketing, Resolutions, and Reference)

MNA's 1985 Legislative Platform stated:

> "MNA advocates enactment and implementation of legislation that will benefit the health and welfare of the nation's citizens and participates in the election of candidates to public office who are knowledgeable about and supportive of the profession."

Legislative goals were identified for these categories: Human Rights, Funding Basic Needs, Health Hazards, Access to Quality Care, Financing Health Care, Funding Nursing Education and Nursing Research, Licensure and Nursing Practice, and Economic and General Welfare of Nursing.

Seeing a need for a united front of nursing professionals showing support for nursing and nursing issues, the MNA Oakland District Legislative Committee, co-chaired by Ann Mentz and Marilyn

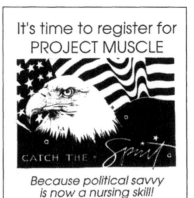

It's time to register for PROJECT MUSCLE

CATCH THE *Spirit*

Because political savvy is now a nursing skill!

Van Tassel, launched the concept of Project MUSCLE. A series of meetings with nurses from other organizations were held at the home of Drs. Bea and Phil Kalisch. As a result, the first Project MUSCLE was held September 21 and 22, 1987 in Lansing. The goal was to bring the voice of the 92,000 registered nurses in Michigan to the State Legislature.

Project MUSCLE evolved into an annual event with some 25 nursing organizations involved, through COMON, the Coalition of Michigan Organizations of Nursing.

With nurses coming together on major issues such as chemical dependency, third party reimbursement, maternal and child services, access to long term care,

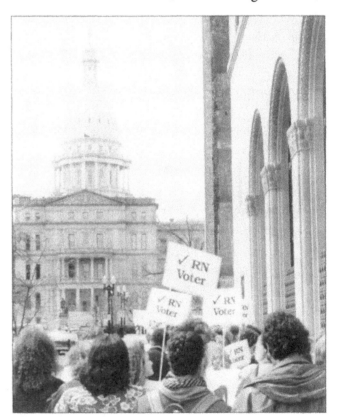

Nursing's annual legislative event (initially known as Project MUSCLE) teaches nurses how to use political power.

immigration nursing relief, tobacco tax proposal, care at the end of life, and the Health Practitioner Recovery Act, the profession began to see progress in moving its issues ahead.

Another strategy to strengthen and unite nursing's voice was MNA's Legislative Committee's establishment of the Legislative Contact Network in 1989. In addition to providing support for the MNA Legislative Platform, members were "to become personally familiar to their legislators as experts on health care who have access to information on the issues which concern the nursing profession." And MNA's political action committee, INPUT (Involved Nurses Politically United Together), changed its name to the straightforward "MNA-PAC (MNA Political Action Committee)."

After much public testimony from MNA leadership and staff, the Board of Nursing proposed rules to establish a system of assessing the continued competence of

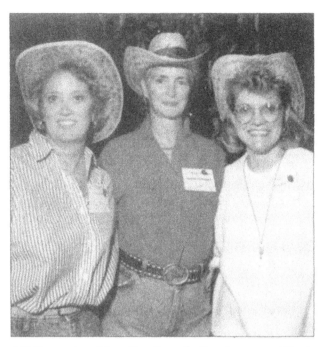

MNA members Mary Fox, Dorothy Pennington and Terrie Ellis, RNs at Bixby Medical Center, donned western garb to join in the line dancing lessons, part of the MNA -PAC fundraising event that drew hundreds of would-be dancers during the convention.

Coalition of Michigan Organizations of Nursing (COMON)

by Jonnie Hamilton, RN, MS

The Coalition of Michigan Organizations of Nursing (COMON) was the brain child of then Michigan Nurses Association President, Dorothea Milbrandt and MNA executive director, Nadine Furlong and was created in the early 1980s. The purpose of COMON was to establish a network of Michigan Nursing Organizations to share information, unify efforts and take action on issues of common concern. Membership was open to all nursing organizations in Michigan and meetings were biannually at the MNA office on Spartan Street in East Lansing. Hosting of meetings was rotated among participating organizations and the meetings were funded by contributions of participants at each meeting.

In 1991 the organization under MNA Executive Director Carol Franck and MNA President Patricia Underwood decided that a more formal organizational process needed to be implemented in order for the coalition to be effective. Bylaws were written with a dues process, officers, and expanded purpose to provide an organized and unified voice for nursing on issues of common concern to intermediaries, legislators and regulatory bodies, to provide for the exchange of appropriate information with those interested in nursing, and to promote understanding, co-operation and communication among nursing organizations.

Those Who Marched
Regina Williams, RN, PhD

by Jess Merrill

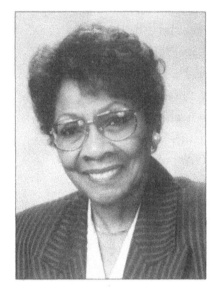

Regina Sallee Williams graduated from Mount Carmel School of Nursing in Columbus, Ohio in 1952 and from Ohio State University in 1955. She subsequently received an MSN from Wayne State University and a PhD degree from the University of Michigan.

Williams can't remember when she did not want to be a nurse. She says, "My grandmother was a practical nurse and a midwife in Kentucky where, I was told, she rode her horse to the homes of women who sent for her to deliver their babies."

Williams began her career in nursing as an operating room nurse. She has been active in the professional association since graduating from nursing. She states, "I was very active with the Ohio State Nurses Association [OSNA], and shortly after we moved to Detroit from Columbus, Ohio in 1966, I became active in the Detroit District of MNA and was a delegate to the MNA conventions. In 1980 I was elected to the MNA Board of Directors. As First Vice President, I chaired the Leadership Development Retreat for two years as the Association leadership developed goals for the organization. In 1983 I was elected MNA President. At that time there were close to 7,000 members in the Association." She served as MNA president from 1983-1985, and she has the distinction of being MNA's first African-American president.

During Williams' tenure as MNA President there were many noteworthy issues and challenges including control of nursing practice, third party reimbursement for nurses in advanced practice and the issue of the baccalaureate degree as the appropriate level of education for entry into nursing practice. There also were intra-organizational issues such as the Association's perceived responsiveness to the membership and to the need for change as well as the issue of the organization's appropriate resource utilization. Legislative issues at the state and national level were important and attention to these issues was fostered by the National Nursing Agenda developed by the ANA. Nurses were exhorted to be "Visible in Politics and Viable in Practice" and to participate in the development of public policy that affected health care.

This was a very busy time for the Association, and, as in all large organizations, it was not without some turmoil. Dr. Williams provided leadership that effectively helped guide the organization through a difficult time by bringing various factions together thus facilitating the organization to move forward.

She said about her career, "If I had it to do over again, I would still choose to become a nurse. It is a very rewarding profession and one that I have participated in and enjoyed for fifty years."

Those Who Marched
Carol E. Franck, RN, MS

by Jess Merrill

Carol E. Franck, RN, MS, chose a career in nursing because of "the great combination of intellectual challenge, and directly making a difference in people's lives." She completed her bachelor's program at Cornell University-New York Hospital School of Nursing in 1960; then moved west to complete a master's degree at the University of California, San Francisco in 1962.

Carol's first nursing position was evening charge nurse on a general surgical floor at New York Hospital, New York, New York. She joined the Michigan Nurses Association in 1970 when she and her family moved to Michigan. Shortly thereafter, she accepted a faculty position in the School of Nursing at Michigan State University where she became known as "compulsively organized and precise."

She joined the staff of MNA as Director of Legislative Affairs in 1984, and in 1986 accepted the position of Executive Director. Carol guided the Association through a great number of changes including the move to a new headquarters building in Okemos. However, she considers her greatest challenges were "to find and maintain the balance among the several membership constituent groups within the organization, and to establish and maintain a stable financial environment within the organization which was well understood by the

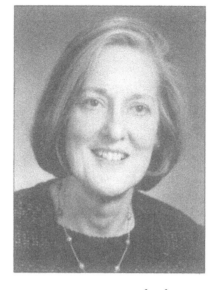

. . . nurses are the best advocates for health care consumers – if only they would realize the leadership they could take and the power they could exert in this arena.

-Carol E. Franck

Board of Trustees and the membership."

Her resolution to both issues was to establish and maintain clear and open communication, and recruit and support staff with the specialized skills needed to accomplish these objectives.

Carol views her most significant contribution to nursing as her commitment to "...advocacy for nurses to policy makers and to other interest groups, and the education of MNA's membership about current issues being debated within the state."

At the end of 1999 Carol resigned her position as Executive Director and retired to Cape Cod where she said, "I intend to become a thorn in the side of the Massachusetts Medical Society whenever I think they need it." While she has done some consulting since leaving MNA, she insists, "I am retired and loving it!"

When asked if she would still choose nursing as a career, she said, "Without question! After all of these years I still see nursing as a great combination of intellectual challenge and directly making a difference in people's lives. And, knowing what I now know, I would add to my original perception the fact that nurses are the best advocates for health care consumers – if only they would realize the leadership they could take and the power they could exert in this arena."

nurses as a condition of license renewal in 1986, requiring 8 hours of continuing education in the previous two years. However, the Board withdrew Competency Rules from the administrative approval process due to a 1988 hiring freeze mandated by the Blanchard administration. It was not until 1997 that mandatory continuing education became a requirement.

The MNA Task Force on Standardization of Nursing Education members Crystal Lange (chairperson), Margo Barron, Julia Stocker, Patricia Lambert, Patricia Underwood, Phyllis Walker, Laurie Weibel, Lynn Moon and Joann Wilcox devoted hours to this issue and in the end recommended that we "must differentiate between the technical and professional practice of nursing." Thus, HB 4911 introduced by Mat Dunaskiss (R-61st district) in 1987, which required a BSN to become licensed as a registered professional nurse after July 1, 1991, was supported by MNA. Key to MNA's support of the bill was the "grandparenting" of all RNs into the registered professional nurse category. The bill created a new category – associate nurse – for nurses educated at the diploma level after 1991, and at the associate degree level after 1996. All LPNs were grandparented into the associate nurse category. While the bill raised significant controversy, it was never voted out of committee.

Governor Engler's signing of the Health Professional Disciplinary Reform legislation, including the Health Professional Recovery Act, on July 8, 1993, marked the culmination of nearly five years of lobbying. The Act changed the way the 15 health profession licensing boards at that time regulated the professions, and changed the disciplinary system. It was estimated in 1989 that one nurse in 50, or 2% of Michigan's 133,000 practicing nurses, were addicted to drugs. Under the revised Public Health Code, which went into effect on April 1, 1994, the Board of Nursing established "a voluntary program which would accept diversion into treatment and voluntary suspension of license during the treatment program as an alternative to disciplinary action." The Act also called for greater

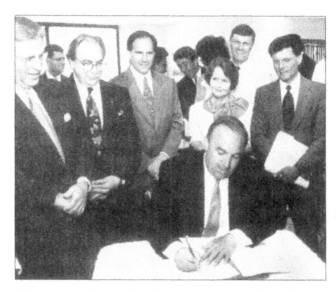

Witnessing Gov. John Engler's signing of the Health Professional Recovery Act in 1993 were (l-r) W. Peter Mccabe, MD, MSMS Board Chair; Eugene Oliversi, DO, Michigan Association of Osteopathic Physicians & Surgeons; Rep. Michael Goschka (R-Saginaw); Patricia Underwood, MNA President; and Sen. John Pridnia (R-Hubbard Lake).

public representation on the boards, and required the mandatory reporting of public health code violations.

A $10 licensure fee increase was included in the reform legislation. As a result of MNA's lobbying efforts, $2 of the annual fees collected from nurses was deposited into a Nurse Professional Fund which provides funding for the establishment and administration of a nursing continuing education program; research to achieve more cost-effective utilization of nurses; and the establishment of nursing scholarships to meet the demands in underserved areas of the state."

The passage of durable power of attorney legislation in 1990, which was first introduced in 1974, was another victory for MNA and the nursing profession. Michigan residents were allowed to give another person the ability to made medical treatment decisions for them should they become incapacitated.

The US focused on Michigan as Dr. Jack Kevorkian made public the issue of physician-assisted suicide and end-of-life issues in general. As a result in 1992, Public Act 270 was passed into law, which made physician-assisted suicide a felony, and created the Commission on Death and Dying. Denise Jacobs, chair of MNA's

Legislative Committee, and Margaret Campbell represented MNA on the Commission, which was charged to "look at the issue of voluntary self-termination of life, with or without assistance." The Determination of Death Act, Public Act 90 of 1992 also passed, which permitted physicians or RNs to pronounce death. According to the August 1992 *Michigan Nurse*, "the language allowing RNs to pronounce death was originated by Mary Lindquist, director of Arbor Hospice in Ann Arbor, in an effort to avoid unwanted resuscitation efforts which can occur upon death in a home, nursing home or hospice residential setting."

A new disease known as AIDS also caused changes in health care regulation. Governor Blanchard signed a package of seven AIDS bills into law at the end of 1988, including a bill that created communicable disease and serious communicable disease categories in the Public Health Code. With this came the mandatory testing of pregnant women for venereal disease, HIV and hepatitis B, a new wave of screening and advising guidelines for healthcare workers, and confidentiality clauses for all the new rules. In June 1989, the Michigan Department of Public Health reported 416 cases of and 167 deaths attributed to AIDS in Michigan during the prior year. For a one-year period (June 1988-May 1989) 91% of the cases were male, 51% white and 46% black, and 43% in their thirties. MNA adopted a Statement of Beliefs at the 1989 HOD, and the December 1989 *Michigan Nurse* was devoted to the topic. Betty J. Beard, PhD, RN, on the Cabinet of Nursing Research, attended the Fourth International Conference on AIDS in Stockholm.

Third Party Reimbursement continued to be a major initiative, building on a 1976 HOD resolution. In 1981 the Joint Committee on Reimbursement (J-CORE) was formed, bringing specialty nursing organizations together with MNA to address the issue. This collaboration resulted in the introduction of a four-bill package introduced by Representative Debbie Stabenow in 1984. Julie Sochalski, PhD, RN, became the first nurse on the Blue Cross/Blue Shield

(BC/BS) of Michigan Board of Directors in October 1986. An additional incremental victory came in 1989 when Attorney General Frank Kelley issued an opinion stating:

> "Blue Cross-Blue Shield of Michigan may not deny reimbursement to a licensed specialty nurse for covered services rendered within the scope of the respective specialty nurse certification and nursing license when such services can be lawfully rendered by the nurse without delegation and supervision of a licensed physician."

In 1993, BC/BS began a pilot program for nurse practitioners preceeded by Medicaid in 1991.

As laws impacting health care were enacted, there was a shortage of nurses, also impacting health care. In 1986 the average starting salary for RNs was $20,340. According to 1987 ANA Executive Director Judith A. Ryan, PhD, RN:

> "The nursing shortage stems from a variety of factors: 1) dramatic changes in the attitudes, values, and aspirations of the potential recruitment pool for nursing; 2) a demo-graphically-driven decline in the number of people entering college; 3) massive changes in the way in which health care is delivered and paid for; and 4) changing roles within the health service sector itself.
>
> The most obvious among these factors, however are the conditions in hospitals within which 68 percent of the estimated 1.5 million working registered nurses practice. Overall these problems in healthcare facilities employing nurses are: 1) modest financial rewards compared with their responsibilities; 2) limited authority for the clinical practice of nursing; and 3) insufficient involvement in hospital management decision regarding standards of nursing practice and essential support services."

MNA President Joann Wilcox provided testimony to the Commission on the Nursing Shortage, part of the US Department of Health and Human Services (HHS), in Chicago on March 7, 1988. It was noted:

"that although HHS has yet to admit that a shortage of nurses does exist, according to the Commission only 23.8 percent of hospitals indicate adequate nurse staffing, and the patient-to-nurse ratio has risen from 50 per 100 patients in 1972 to 50 per 191 patients in 1986."

A 1989 survey of 131 chief executive officers and nursing executives in Michigan revealed a 9.82% RN vacancy rate and a 12.42% RN turnover rate, with an average of 11.4 weeks needed to fill a medical/surgical position and 15.6 weeks to fill an ICU/CCU position.

The Michigan Department of Public Health Advisory Task Force on Nursing Issues, chaired by Dr. Gloria Smith, reported in May of 1990 that "the nursing shortage in Michigan was a chronic and growing problem, particularly in specialized fields, and needs to be addressed with better pay for experienced nurses, more options for independent practice and a new state office to coordinate state policies to better develop the profession."

Intern/extern programs, retention of specialists and researchers, differentiated practice and scholarships and loans were also part of the Michigan strategy. Retention rates did increase as hospitals improved working conditions and benefits, some voluntarily and some as a result of collective bargaining agreements. At Pontiac General Hospital flexible shifts were implemented, and nurses who worked three 12-hour shifts earned full-time health care and holiday benefits. E.W. Sparrow Hospital in Lansing and Sinai Hospital in Detroit recognized nurses who work permanent weekends to be full-time employees. The University of Michigan Hospitals changed their hour shift differential and added yearly bonuses, with the result being that 250 nurses signed up for permanent off-shift positions in the two months following this change. Borgess Hospital became the first hospital to implement a shared governance model that provided staff nurses a voice in decisions that affected their patients and the work environment.

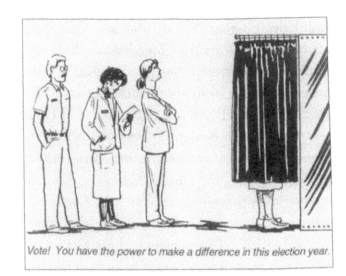

Vote! You have the power to make a difference in this election year.

Health care reform became a familiar phrase in the early 90s as work began on *Nursing's Agenda for Health Care Reform*, and nurses were encouraged to become politically active and vote!

MNA's Health Care Reform Task Force began to look at President Clinton's health care reform package – the American Health Security Act of 1993 – which drew interest from nurses across the country and was the focus of the October 1993 issue of *Michigan Nurse*. With health promotion, disease prevention and primary care at its core, it promised to increase the role of nurses, nurse midwives and other health care professionals in primary and preventative care. The package reflected many nurses' views, in that problems of inadequate access, sky-rocketing costs, and improving quality must all be addressed.

Changes in labor law also greatly influenced MNA's E&GW program and organizing efforts. In 1974 RN-only units were considered appropriate. In the early 1980s the National Labor Relations Board (NLRB) changed its attitude and in 1984 decided that RN-only units were not appropriate. However, in 1991 the Supreme Court ruled in favor of RN-only bargaining units in a case a hospital brought against the NLRB.

Nurses across the state voted for MNA representation as working conditions worsened. The Sparrow Hospital organizing campaign was launched during this time when RN-only units were deemed inappropriate. This campaign was a multi-union effort, with MNA organizing the professional staff, including the RNs, and the other unions working to organize the service/maintenance employees, and the technical/clerical employees, including licensed practice nurses.

Nurses at Allegan General and North Ottawa Hospitals both selected MNA as their representative in 1988. Ontonagon Memorial Hospital RNs organized in January of 1991 because of concerns about wages and patient care. The Lapeer Regional Hospital RNs became the first collective bargaining unit organized after the Supreme Court ruled in April of that year "that registered nurses are an appropriate unit in and of themselves for purposes of elections and collective bargaining."

As the E&GW program matured and gains were being made, the issue of "should professional nurses be represented through collective bargaining" was again raised. Jody Berney, RN, chairperson of the E&GW Cabinet in 1991 wrote:

> "By the mid '80s, increasing numbers of nurses found that the collective bargaining option could help them to improve their wages and their working conditions. Recognizing this, other traditional labor unions began to focus their attentions on members of our profession as well...It is of critical importance that we understand why nurses choose MNA. There is simply no substitute for our professional association. The nurses organized with MNA believe that nurses must control nursing...No other labor union has the tradition of practice issues addressed in contract language as well as MNA...Let us stand together to face the challenge ahead of us and to help us remain the voice of nursing in this state."

A sampling of contracts show MNA continued to make economic and practice gains for nurses through collective bargaining. The Calhoun County Health Department RNs negotiated a nine percent wage increase. Macomb County Health Department RNs

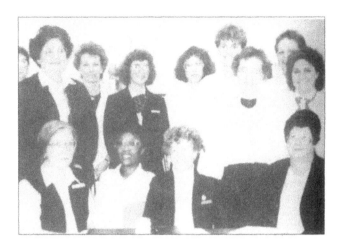

Calhoun County members enjoy a quiet moment after negotiations. (Front l-r) Barb Pipley, Sarita Williams, Sue Siddall, Sara Robertson. (Center l-r) Joyce Henderson, Phyllis Killian, Joyce Ann Murphy, Julie Shippy. (Back l-r) Martha Myers, Diane Bunch, Pat Bradley, Dianne Niecko and Ella Mauer.

successfully bargained to continue to receive free hepatitis B shots despite the county's demand that the nurses pay a fee. Martha T. Berry Medical Care Facility RNs improved their sick-leave and created a permanent panel of arbitrators to hear disputes.

Not all gains were made easily. In 1989, the nursing shortage took its toll at University of Michigan Medical Center where the University of Michigan Professional Nurse Council (UMPNC) members struck over mandatory overtime and issues of patient care.

In 1990, Borgess Medical Center nurses protested unilateral changes in their prescription benefits by signing grievances and threatening to establish informational picketing. The Crittenton Hospital nurses had three nurse agencies break the picket line during their strike, which prompted MNA to call on ANA to create an effective national policy towards strike breaking nurses.

After two years without a contract and a year after they officially issued a work stoppage notice, Saginaw County Health Department RNs staged the first public health nurse strike in Michigan in October 1991. And Allegan General Hospital RNs were on strike for 14 days over the nurses' right to maintain 12-hour shifts.

Professional Employee Council of Sparrow Hospital

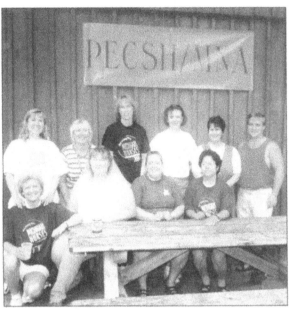

PECSH team: (Back row l-r) – Kathy Dunn, RN, Deb Walde, RN, Diane Goddeeris, RN, Joanne Polanski, RN, Jessica Salazar, MNA labor representative, and Jeff Breslin, RN. (Front row l-r) – Gail Jehl, RN, Deb Bearup, RN, Gail Fisher, RN, and Jesusa Vasquez, RN.

By Gail Jehl, RN

The employees of E.W. Sparrow Hospital organized its local bargaining unit, PECSH in 1987 with a certification election by the National Labor Relations Board (NLRB). The PECSH membership ratified its first collective bargaining agreement October 31, 1988 after a lengthy negotiating process with Sparrow Hospital administration.

The organizing effort was slow and tedious. Hospital administration provided an issue that gave the process a jump start, late in 1986. Sparrow management celebrated navigating the new DRG reimbursement process by purchasing and providing top level administration with company vehicles. On Mother's Day 1986 they announced the unpaid lunch period would be increased from ½ hour to 1 full hour for all RNs; reducing the number of paid work hours. This was a significant loss of wages – from two to five hours each pay period. This reduction of hours paid was the final motivation needed for successful local unit organizing.

Sparrow management attempted to dilute the organizing effort by requesting all health care professionals be included in the bargaining unit. The NLRB ruled that all non-management employees with a Bachelors degree or higher and all non-management RNs would be included in the unit. With the successful NLRB election, the PECSH local was formed and included approximately 40 different classifications. These classifications include registered nurses, physical therapists, speech therapists, occupational therapists, medical technologists, pharmacists, social workers, dieticians and many more.

The first years were growing years for the PECSH local unit. One person often filled multiple roles. The following people have served or are currently serving on the executive council: Office of chairperson; Deloris Pyleman, Deb Stevens, Terri Peaphon, Cathy Dunn and Kimberly Ford. Office of vice-chairperson; Kathy Boyton, Linda Makela, Jesusa Vasquez, Margaret Flynn and Diane Goddeeris. Grievance chairperson; Bob Ehnis, Terri Peaphon, Douglas Church, Jesusa Vasquez, Gail Jehl. Recording secretary; Suzanne Allen, Rita Michaels, Jesusa Vasquez, Tania Atwood. Treasurer; Bob Ehnis, Jeffrey Holiday, and Judy McLane. Health Professional Representative; Sally Chirio, Gordon Taylor, and Jackie Walker. Under this leadership a strong base of support has been established.

Building a strong labor/management partnership became a priority in 1995. Executive council members, negotiating committee members, and MNA representatives along with Sparrow Human Resources and the management team representatives attended several forms of training to begin developing a cooperative relationship that would prove mutually beneficial. Site visits to the Saturn Corporation, Work in America Institute and work with Michigan State University and The National Center for Dispute Settlement (NCDS) took place over several years.

A merger with St. Lawrence Hospital took place between 1997 and 1998. All professional employees at St. Lawrence were incorporated into the PECSH local unit. A short term contract was negotiated that addressed many of the transition issues of the merger along with wages, seniority and work reassignments. Lori Certo was appointed to serve as the St. Lawrence representative to our executive team during this period. The transition was successfully accomplished without any professional staff being laid off.

PECSH has successfully negotiated six contracts with Sparrow Hospital. In addition to wage and benefit increases, we obtained unit specific staffing levels in 1994 and language that allows for changes in staffing levels through a mutual gains process. Members have direct input _and_ approval of changes that affect their work related to staffing. In 200l, we gained language that prohibits the use of mandatory overtime. The current contract expires on October 31, 2004.

The 2003 PECSH leadership is comprised of seasoned representatives and newly involved activists. They continue to promote and advocate for nursing and all other represented professionals. Many of the current leadership participate in Michigan Nurses Association (MNA) at the state level. Kimberly Ford, PECSH chairperson serves on the Economic and General Welfare (E&GW) Cabinet. Diane Goddeeris currently serves as

PECSH vice-chairperson and also the Chapter VI representative to the MNA Board of Directors. Gail Jehl, grievance chairperson, E&GW representative to the MNA Board of Directors and also serves on the Congress for Nursing Practice. Previous leaders have built on their experience in PECSH, including Terri Peaphon who joined the MNA staff as a Labor Organizer in 1999.

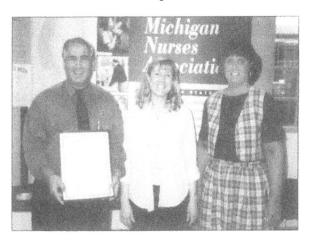

(l-r) MNA Associate Executive Director of Labor Relations John Karebian, Kathy Dunn, RN, and PECSH Chairperson Kimberly Ford, RN display a Nurses Week proclamation at the MNA/PECSH booth.

Several PECSH members have received the prestigious E&GW achievement award; Bob Ehnis, Terri Peaphon, Jesusa Vasquez, Gail Jehl, Diane Goddeeris and Kimberly Ford have been recognized for their contributions to building a strong and cohesive union at Sparrow.

PECSH Mission Statement

The Professional Employee Council of Sparrow Hospital (PECSH) shall be the powerful, effective, unified force, working together to provide the highest quality patient care and optimal working conditions.

As equal partners, the membership will collaborate in the planning and decision making related to delivery of care and the well being of the PECSH membership.

Our strength is in individual members uniting to support each other in this mission.

Lapeer Registered Nurse Staff Council

The Lapeer Registered Nurse Staff Council at Lapeer Regional Hospital was started around 1989, after management announced major changes in the health care benefits. Mary Kozik, RN, an ICU nurse, contacted MNA on behalf of all RNs. Betty Dice, Mary Kozik, Judy Johnston, Penny Gates and a few others worked on organizing and getting cards signed. After the vote was won came the long struggle to get a first contract. Negotiations started in February 1992 and continued through April 30, 1993. The first contract was ratified and went into effect May 9, 1993. During the first negotiations, a small group of nurses attempted to decertify the union, which resulted in a second vote. MNA was again selected to represent the registered nurses.

In 1999, while attempting to gain improvements with the third contract reopener, negotiations failed. Nurses struck over unfair labor practices and overtime. The strike lasted about 14

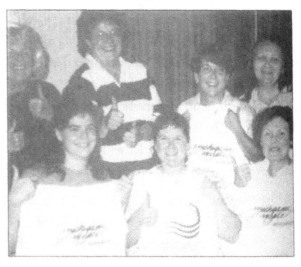

Lapeer Regional Hospital Organizing Committee members celebrate their September 12, 1991 election for MNA representation.

days. Betty Dice was the first President from 1990 through 1999. Her successors were Leigh Childers, Barb Woolard, and Penny Gates (the current President). In May 2003, nurses ratified their fourth contract which some believe to be our best yet. Currently 140 RNs are represented by MNA.

Marquette General RNs reached their 1991 agreement, giving them a 22 percent wage increase over three years, just hours before a strike deadline. "They insisted that their wages and benefits were not the proper target for cost-cutting, citing the growing responsibility of RNs for patient care and the steady market for their services."

As the demand for collective bargaining services increased, so did the need for office facilities. The MNA board had approved the sale of MNA's Spartan Avenue building in East Lansing and the search was on for a new location at their January 1990 meeting. The Building Replacement Task Force consisting of Toni Stevenson, Sandra Fritz-Kelly, Nannette Bills and Lillian Simms went to work to find a new building site, review numerous specifications, and make all the internal material selections. The decision was made to build in a new professional park being

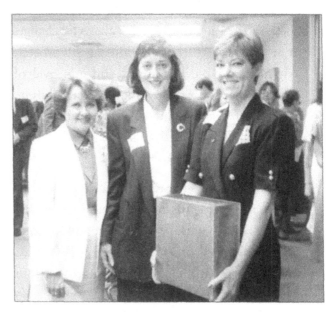

MNA President Pat Underwood, Executive Director Carol Franck, and Building Replacement Task Force Chair Toni Stevenson prepare to place the time capsule during MNA's open house celebrating their new headquarters.

developed called Okemos + Oak Park, near the Okemos Road exit off of I-96. The "Nursing on the Move; 1990-1991 Capital Campaign" was launched in the fall of 1990 and the move into MNA's current headquarters occurred on March 1, 1991, right on schedule. An Open House was held on July 17 and a time capsule was placed in the cornerstone, commemorating the occasion.

Nurses Week was commemorated annually, and the District-level Nurses Week celebrations were as varied as the districts. In 1998, Barry-Calhoun District offered a full-day presentation and a book-signing reception with author Melodie Chenevert, RN, MSN. Grand Rapids District had a luncheon and program featuring Marcia Anderson, RN, PhD, President of Personalized Nursing Corporation. Lenawee District held a health care forum with Representative Tim Walberg, Senator Norman Shinke and Jim Berryman. Sault Sainte Marie District honored nurse anthropologist, Dee Light as their Nurse of the Year. The Capital Area District's dinner and program featured Julie Sochalski, RN, PhD, a senior policy analyst with Pro-Pac. Her topic was "Sleeping Giants: Motivating Nurses to be Politically Active." And, Miss American 1988, Kaye Lani Rae Rafko, RN, joined the Wayne County Professional Nurses' Council celebration.

In 1989 the *Michigan Nurse* devoted an entire page of the April issue to encourage Michigan nurses to "Nix the Nightingales." To quote the article introduction: "The steamy image of nursing presented in NBC's Nightingales (Wednesday at 10:00 p.m.) has prompted many complaints from nurses about the show's bimbos-over-brains approach." It was noted that Chrysler, Sears and McDonalds had announced plans to pull their ads. The advertisers that had not done so were listed, along with contact information. Shortly after, NBC cancelled the show, deciding "the controversy around the show was too great to renew it for a second season."

Liz Galvin reported that members of the Detroit District Nurses Association, their friends and families,

Those Who Marched
Kay Lani Rae Rafko, RN

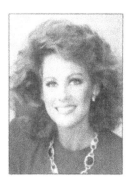

Needing to finance her nursing education, Kaye Lani Rae Rafko entered a beauty contest – and won. The former Miss Lapeer County and Miss Michigan ultimately won the Miss America 1988 contest.

During her year of service and afterward, Kaye Lani advocated for nursing and hospice programs. Her social activism so impressed pageant officials that they developed an official platform to permit contest winners to promote worthy causes and be role models for public service.

Following her reign as Miss America, Kaye Lani opened a hospice program in Monroe. She has addressed many national organizations and medical professional groups worldwide about nursing and health care issues, including cancer and AIDS.

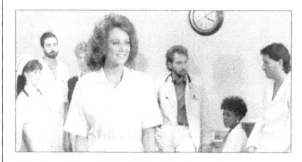

Kaye Lani Rae Rafko, RN, Miss America 1988, tapes a public service announcement, "Proud to Care," created to encourage young people to choose nursing as a career.

participated in the "Relay for Life", September 16-17, sponsored by the American Cancer Society.

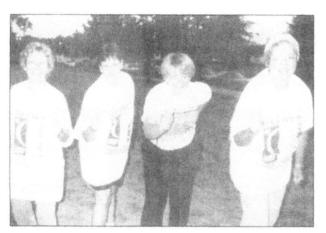

Detroit District team members Ramona Benkert, Judy McCornish, Elizabeth Galvin and Sharolyn White get ready for the American Cancer Society's annual fundraising event.

And as this decade came to an end, somber moments mingled with the occasions for celebration. MNA members honored their nurse colleagues who had served in the armed services with a raffle for the Vietnam Women's Memorial Project which raised $3,700. MNA board member Sandie Wilson, a Vietnam veteran, was the major force behind the fundraising. First prize, a limited edition miniature of a statue titled "Nurse" (right) went to Sue Bennett of Ann Arbor. Sandie Wilson, and fellow nurse veteran and MNA member Peggy Flatt attended the unveiling ceremony on November 11, 1993.

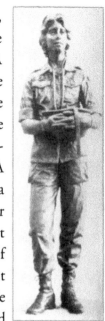

1994-2003

by Ann Sincox and Carol Feuss

The New Millennium, Terrorists Strike the US, and a Nursing Shortage

The final decade of the Michigan Nurses Association's first 100 years as the voice for registered nurses in Michigan was stunning for the world in many areas. Technology shrank as pocket organizers gained the ability to access the Internet without wires, and compact discs (CD) minimized full-length movies and music onto DVDs (Digital Video Disk). Small cloned cells turned into a full size Scottish sheep named Dolly, and cyberspace grew into the use of virtual reality. Small bits of punched-out paper called hanging chads left a Presidential election upside down as a few hundred votes (and 60 days of recounting ballots) decided between George Bush or Al Gore winning the Presidency. Stem cell research is seen as a potential source of help for several diseases, including Alzheimer's, and the use of DNA as a forensic tool is popularized in television shows *CSI, CSI: Miami* and *CSI: New York*. The highly anticipated "Millenium Bug," which threatened to create chaos as computers supposedly couldn't read "2000" as the world entered the new century turned out to be nothing more than a sniffle.

Infectious diseases continue to travel easily over borders and have international officials searching for answers as SARS (Severe Acute Respiratory Syndrome) appeared in the Orient and traveled to Canada and the United States in 2003. Although tuberculosis, rampant and virulent 100 years ago is considered under control in developed countries, in 1998 there were 35 countries with a newer, drug-resistant strain. A type of mosquito carrying the West Nile virus has been rough on the elderly with 2001-2004 marked as epidemic years. And HIV-AIDS continues its deadly toll, with 100 million estimated deaths at the end of 2003 in Russia alone.

Unfortunately, 1994-2004 brought the ugly reality of terrorism to Americans, both inside and outside our national borders. On August 19, 1995, a homemade bomb in a rented truck destroyed half of the Murrah Federal Building in Oklahoma City, OK, killing 168 persons and injuring over 500. Timothy McVeigh was executed on June 11, 2001 for the bombing, with his ex-Army friend Terry Nichols, a Michigan resident, receiving life imprisonment. One year later, a homemade pipe bomb was detonated near the main Olympic sites in Atlanta, GA, killing one person and causing a photojournalist to die of a heart attack while fleeing the scene.

It was on September 11, 2001, however, that the world watched in horror as four hijacked domestic airplanes crashed into the World Trade Center buildings in New York, the Pentagon in Washington, DC, and a Pennsylvania field. Nurses swarmed to the hospitals and crash sites, offering help and care wherever they could. Sadly, there were many more fatalities than survivors.

While the heart of nursing remained the same, the environment in which nurses practiced and the issues surrounding nursing continued to be altered.

Comprehensive health care reform was exchanged for incremental reform, and the focus shifted from the national to the state level. Hospitals set out to cut costs by massive restructuring and eliminating patient care positions – including registered nurses. MNA's biggest bargaining unit was not immune from the sweeping trend of cutting nursing positions, as the University of Michigan Hospitals announced significant layoffs in 1996.

MNA, as part of a $5 million US Department of Labor grant to develop a retraining program for dislocated health care workers, undertook the task of helping nurses make the transition into the growing number of ambulatory care positions created as a result of the restructuring.

Perhaps more than any other nursing specialty, psychiatric/mental health nurses experienced great turmoil as their practice moved out of institutions and community-based practice became the norm. A statewide re-education program was launched, in collaboration with the Michigan Department of Mental Health, to assist nurses to make the transition from their current inpatient practice area to outpatient

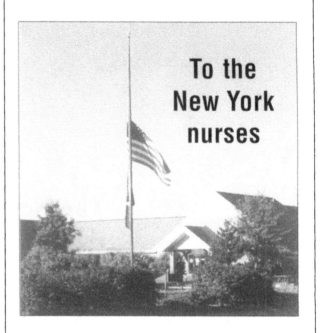

To the New York nurses

We remember . . .

That you were on the front lines,
setting up portable triage units
and swallowing your grief and shock;

That you had loved ones
to worry about, too, yet you stayed;

That you worked until you dropped,
and then got up and worked some more.
The idea of "working a shift"
never crossed your mind;

That you will still be there,
healing the physical and mental scars
long after the TV cameras have gone
and the world has moved on;

Do not think for a moment
that your sacrifice has gone unnoticed.

You are now, and continue to be,
in our hearts.

We are so very proud of you.

Source: *Michigan Nurse*, October, 2001
Author: Ann Kettering Sincox

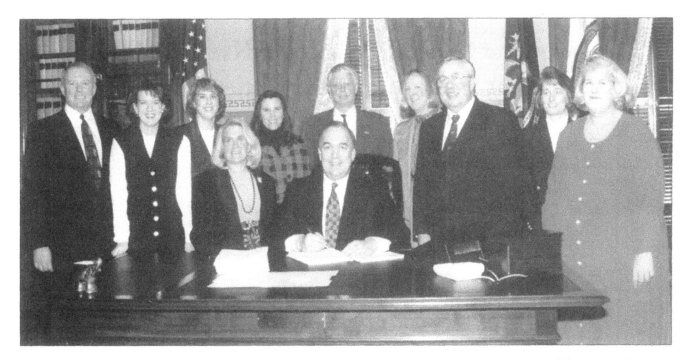

Governor Engler signs the newly revised State of Michigan Mental Health Code, 1996. Center of front row (l-r) Rep. Beverly Hammerstrom, House Mental Health Policy Committee Chair, Governor John Engler, and Senator Joel Gougeon, Chair, Senate Mental Health Policy Committee. Center of back row: Deborah Bach Coley, MNA Director of Government Affairs; Jim Haveman, Director of Michigan Department of Community Health; and Andrea Bostrom, Member, MNA Psychiatric Nursing Practice Committee. The three additional people on the left and the two on the right are staff of mental health programs and legislative offices. MNA took an active role in advocating for patient rights and proper acknowledgement of the role of the professional nurse and advanced practice psychiatric nurse in the 1995-96 revisions to the Michigan Mental Health Code, and Governor Engler invited the MNA member and staff representatives from the Mental Health Code Workgroups to the bill signing.

psychiatric/mental health nursing. Over 325 RNs attended the educational sessions in 1995. MNA was instrumental in the rewriting of the Michigan Mental Health Code, which recognized nurses as "Mental Health Professionals" and included nurses in expanded areas of practice. The code became law effective March 27, 1996.

The January 1998 *Michigan Nurse* reminded members there are "many issues to consider in today's changing health care systems." MNA created a "Position Statement on Mergers, Acquisitions, Affiliations, Collaborative Arrangements and Joint Ventures" which articulated principles to guide discussions. Visible in the conversation was the issue of profit vs not-for-profit hospitals, although all Michigan hospitals today remain not-for-profit corporations.

Yet another outcome of the fluctuating environment was concerns for patients' safety, which escalated to

national attention. MNA members joined more than 25,000 nurse colleagues to protest unsafe patient care in hospitals during the ANA co-sponsored "Nurses March in Washington" in 1995. The Institute of Medicine issued a series of reports identifying concerns within health systems in general, and focusing on medical errors. The Michigan Health and Safety Coalition formed in 1999 to address these concerns at the state level. MNA and other associations representing the health care professions, along with industry and consumer representatives, are part of the Coalition. In MNA's centennial year, MNA successfully introduced the Safe Patient Care legislation to eliminate mandatory overtime and establish minimum nurse to patient staffing ratios.

There was much unrest as staff councils were caught in the current of changing systems. Marquette General RNs saw their 1994 contract voted down, and 320

Marquette General Hospital RNs strike for patient safety and better patient care

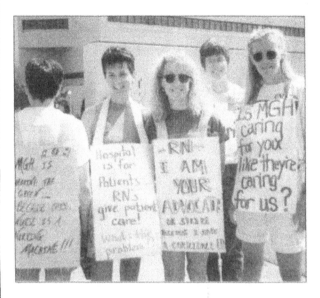

RNs Michelle Johnson, Alison Amundsen, Michele Fonts, Sue Milner and Julie Sharp are five of 320 RNs who went on strike in August, 1994 against Marquette General Hospital.

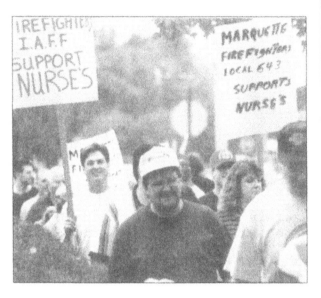

In a show of solidarity, about 2,000 members from 10 Marquette-area unions surrounded Marquette General Hospital September 14 to support striking RNs. The United Steelworkers of America organized the protest after learning that hospital officials threatened to hire permanent replacement nurses.

were on the picket lines for 56 days. The major concern was patient safety and patient care when the hospital was reducing the number of RNs. Key to the settlement was "the creation of a committee of five union RNs and five management RNs to select a system for determining staffing levels within individual hospital units."

Mid-Michigan Health Department nurses rallied together in September 1995 after going seven months without a contract. That same month, MNA represented members employed with the Visiting Nurses Association of Southeast Michigan, who, worried about patient safety, issued a strike notice.

Later that year, RNs at St. Francis Hospital in Escanaba launched an effort to organize, but were initially thwarted by the hospital's position that all RNs are supervisors. Registered nurses at Michigan Capital Medical Center were fighting this same battle in 1994, and MNA intervened on behalf of the nurses as they

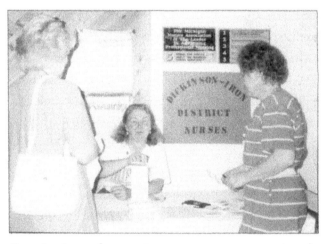

Even in times of uncertainty, nurses were out serving the community. Nurses from the Dickinson-Iron District were active in the 1996 Birchwood Mall Health Fair in Kingsford. Health fair participants received MNA pens and pins and the pamphlet, "Every Patient Deserves a Nurse."

fought the employer's argument "that all the staff nurses were supervisors by virtue of their direction of LPNs and aides." The employers were referring to a

1994 US Supreme Court decision that nurses who direct the work of other employees could potentially be deemed supervisors under federal labor law. This ruling deprived RNs of collective bargaining rights and other workplace protections and was in conflict with another recent ruling that RNs could organize. The nurses appealed to the National Labor Relations Board which ruled in 1996 that all RNs are not supervisors. Their initial election was not successful, however, the RNs launched a new campaign and were victorious in 2003, becoming MNA's 51st bargaining unit.

There were also many gains by nurses represented by MNA during this decade. Hackley Hospital, organized in 1994, was the first hospital whose contract included staffing ratios in their agreement. Sparrow Hospital Professional Employee Staff Council negotiated "unprecedented rights regarding staffing levels and patient safety" in their 1995 contract. The contract ensured "that employees are involved in all decisions regarding staffing levels and skill mix, as well as in the evaluation of future staffing projections and patient acuity system."

MNA's leadership in collective bargaining agreements was demonstrated again in 1999. Nurses at Borgess Medical Center in Kalamazoo, North Ottawa Community Hospital in Grand Haven, and Lapeer Regional Hospital in Lapeer were three of the first nursing groups in the country to negotiate language into their collective bargaining agreements that includes patient protections and disclosure of staffing and outcome data. Lapeer RNs went on strike in order to gain this language.

MNA's two largest bargaining units, Professional Employees Council of Sparrow Hospital and the University of Michigan Professional Nurse Council, were both successful in breaking the $30/hour barrier for registered nurses. They were the first unions in Michigan to do so.

Marquette General Hospital RNs' 2001 contract included a committee to review and recommend a needleless system and a latex-free environment. RNs

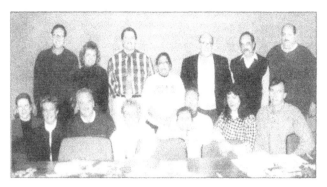

Borgess Medical Center bargaining team celebrated a new two-year contract in 1997. Pictures are (standing l-r): Jim Magnuson, Cheryl West, Pete Krueger, Aydda Aguillar, Craig Miller, Larry Cross, Rick Rich; (kneeling): Heather Hudson, Pat Berger, Dennis Bertch, Cheryl McKee, Helen Hicks, Dennis Lancaster, Gaylia Hanson, and Chris Longton.

at Hackley Hospital made substantial gains in their 2002 contract with the addition of three benefits impacting retirement: a pension plan, and a 403B contribution plan, and a medical reimbursement account usable in retirement.

The demand from nurses for MNA assistance grew as the healthcare system continued to convulse. A 1999 ANA grant enabled the organizing program to expand. In the year that followed, West Shore Hospital RNs, who decertified with another union so they could be represented by MNA, voted for MNA representation in December of 1999. This vote was followed by Iron County Community Hospital voting for MNA in September 2000, and Sturgis Hospital in November 2000.

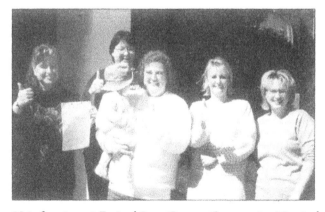

V is for victory! Excited Iron County Community Hospital nurses are celebrating their successful vote to have MNA represent their professional concerns as a collective bargaining agent.

United American Nurses

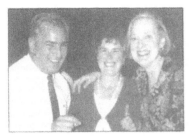

Jubilant MNA staff members celebrate the formation of the United American Nurses, a national nurses union. Pictured are John Karebian, Terri Peaphon and Carol Franck.

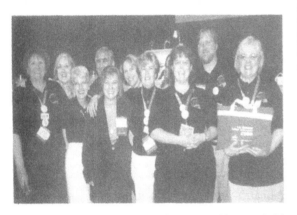

The first UAN National Labor Assembly was held June, 2000. Pictured here are UAN delegates and MNA staff members: (l-r): Carolyn Hietamaki, Carol Franck, Linda Canfield, John Karebian, UAN president Cheryl Johnson, Katy Oppenheim, Terri Pephon, Kris Michaelson, Sharon Anderson, Mark Carlson, and Lisa Mitchem.

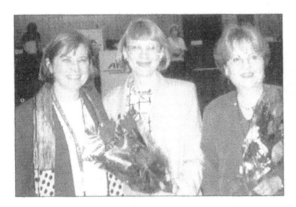

Following her election as the inaugural UAN President, Cheryl Johnson, RN (l) shares a moment with Christina Sieloff, RN, MSN, PhD, ANA Director at Large (c) and Patricia Underwood, RN, PhD, ANA First Vice President (r).

And, in this context, the ANA Economic and General Welfare Program reached the 50 year mark and looked for a change. It began when MNA, with Illinois, Massachusetts, Minnesota, New York, Ohio, Oregon, Washington, and the District of Columbia worked together to create the State Nurses Association Labor Coalition in 1998. Another step came in 1999, as the United American Nurses (UAN) was created as the labor arm of ANA and MNA member Cheryl Johnson was selected as the inaugural President. The headline in the August 1999 *Michigan Nurse* reads: "Michigan delegation helps create new national nurses union." The article begins:

> "Nurses represented for collective bargaining in Michigan and nationally won a significant victory at the ANA House of Delegates in Washington, DC in June. Representatives from the state Nurses Association Labor Coalition initiated the development of a comprehensive plan for a new national nurses union…within the ANA structure."

The succeeding ANA conventions and UAN National Labor Assemblies have continued to address ANA and UAN bylaws as the relationship between the organizations evolve.

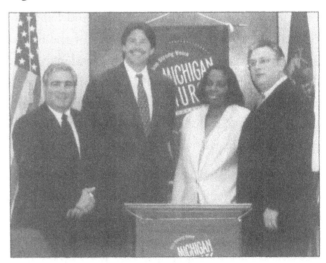

MNA and Michigan AFL-CIO held a joint press conference on May 9, 2001 after the AFL-CIO Executive Council approved the UAN charter. Pictured are: MNA Chief Labor Officer John Karebian, MNA CEO Tom Renkes, Michigan State AFL-CIO Secretary/Treasurer Tina Abbott and Michigan State AFL-CIO President Mark Gaffney.

The UAN was granted a charter by the AFL-CIO in 2001, allowing UAN nurses to join forces with the 13 million members of AFL-CIO to advocate for better patient care, respect, and working conditions for nursing. The national affiliation opened the door for MNA's state-level affiliation later that year.

The turbulence created by change in health care systems impacted all other aspects of nursing as well. Nursing leaders in Michigan also launched a Nursing Futures Initiative to address the "lack of cohesiveness between nursing education and nursing practice. Mary Wawrzynski, PhD, MSN, RN, reported in the May 1996 *Michigan Nurse* that over 100 nurses participated in six regional work groups. The work groups brought together representatives from practice and education, chief nursing officers from small and large hospitals and dean/directors and students from many types of nursing education programs. The outcome of this three year project guided further changes in both the practice and educational systems, and emphasized the essential component of collaboration across fields.

MNA worked to ensure that the voice of nursing was heard over the din of everything else. Nursing's voice was strengthened as Project MUSCLE, the annual nurses lobby day facilitated by MNA and the Coalition of Michigan Organizations of Nursing, became Nurses Impact in 1995. And, impact they had.

MNA began a long legislative road in 1996 when, as part of the Advanced Practice Nurses Coalition

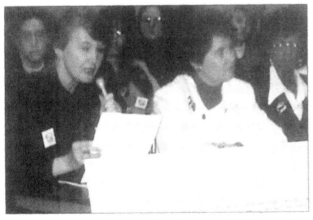

Nursing school deans Marilyn Rothert (MSU) and Ada Sue Hinshaw (U of M) testify in support of prescriptive authority for advanced practice nurses.

(APNC), they were successful in getting legislation introduced to give advanced practice nurses the ability to write prescriptions independent of a physician. This bill made it as far as a committee hearing in 1996 and an identical bill was introduced in 1997. After over a year of discussions, and amendments being accepted, SB 104 passed out of the Senate with a last-minute addition: "only under the supervision of a physician." According to the April 1999 Issue Update in the *Michigan Nurse* "...the prescribing in SB 104 lost all independence and became something MNA could not support. SB 104 died at the end of the session on December, 1998."

APNs made some gains at the national level when the "Primary Care Health Practitioner Incentive Act of 1997," removed geographic restrictions for Medicare reimbursement of advance practice nurses, but kept the payment to NPs and CNSs at 85% of the physician fee schedule for services which they are authorized to perform under state law.

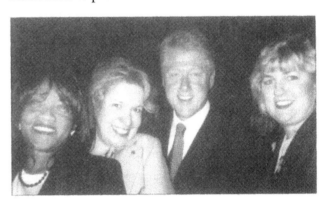

Deb Griffin, MNA president Kimberly Hickey, and Cynthia Gerstenlauer pose with President Clinton at the 1999 Medicare town hall meeting.

Nurses were heard when President Bill Clinton held a town hall style meeting in Lansing in 1999 to discuss his economically-driven Medicare reform proposal. MNA members Cynthia Gerstenlauer, Deb Griffin, MNA president Kimberly Hickey, Jeanette Klemczak, Karen Risch, and Lynn Swick, as well as MNA Director of Government Affairs Judy Pendergast attended this invitation-only event.

Growing concern over blood borne pathogens led to MNA's push for "needle stick" legislation in 1999.

Michigan nurses shared how devastating a needle stick was to their lives and careers, as they testified in support of proposed Michigan legislation. Before the Michigan legislation made it through the entire process, federal rule changes made the legislation unnecessary. The November 2000 passage of federal legislation changed the Occupational Safety and Health Administration (OSHA) standards to require sharps with engineered sharps injury protection features and needleless systems.

In March of 2001, MNA worked with the Michigan Board of Nursing to pass a resolution stating that, "Nurses who refuse to work mandatory overtime, based on their professional judgment, can't be charged with patient abandonment." This was reiterated in a June opinion by then Attorney General Jennifer Granholm. Subsequently, the 2002 MNA House of Delegates passed a resolution reaffirming "its stance against mandatory overtime and asserted its commitment to battle against the continued use of it as a staffing solution." Several bills were introduced in 2004 to eliminate mandatory overtime.

The close of 2002 brought new legislation to protect health care workers who "blow the whistle" on their employers when they see unsafe practices. "We are pleased our government leaders have taken this strong stance to protect quality patient care. Obviously, with more than 100,000 registered nurses in Michigan, it is essential that RNs are able to speak up on behalf of their patient without fearing for their jobs," said MNA president Marylee Pakieser in an MNA press release. Prior to this legislation, nurses were protected only in the case of reporting illegal activities.

A *Michigan Nurse* article by Deborah Coley explains why MNA was effective in many legislative initiatives:

"MNA and other health care professionals met with representatives of the Michigan Department of Commerce, the chairs of the relevant House and Senate committees, and other important and influential members in both houses. The strategy proved to be a classic

example of the value of the efforts of MNA on behalf of nurses in Michigan. Nurses' interests were represented in the process, nurses took a "front and center" leadership role, and nurses were able to build bridges with other associations, legislators and their professional staff."

MNA's Political Action Committee (PAC) grew and expanded its influence. The December 1998 *Michigan Nurse* reports:

"MNA-PAC achieved a 100 percent success rate in getting MNA-supported candidates elected to office when sixty-six new members were elected to the Michigan Legislature. The 1999 House of Delegates approved an increase in the monthly PAC contribution to $1.66/member/month to further strengthen MNA-PAC's position and ensure nurses are heard. The PAC Leadership Circles were created in 2000 to recognize contributors at varying levels, ranging from the Lillian Wald Circle at $100-249 to the Florence Nightingale Circle for contributions of $1,000 or more."

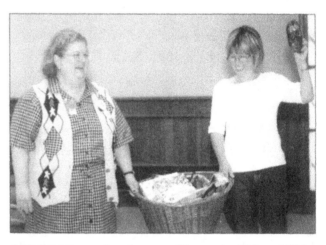

MNA-PAC member Jeanette Klemczak, RN and Terry Smith-Seaver, RN accept bids on a goodie basket for the MNA-PAC auction during Convention 2002.

Recognizing that MNA's continued success required a new look at how things were done, a major restructuring of MNA was undertaken under the direction of MNA President Linda Mondeaux and Executive Director Carol Franck. A long-term strategic plan was developed in 1996, followed by the 1997 MNA House of Delegates approval

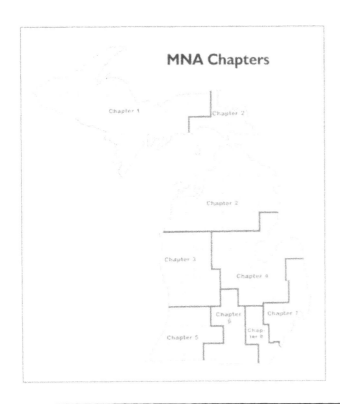

MNA Chapters

Chapter 1

Chapter 2

Chapter 2

Chapter 3

Chapter 4

Chapter 6

Chapter 7

Chap-
ter 8

Chapter 5

of a new structure. Practice Sections were grouped into three Congresses – Nursing Practice, Public Policy, and Nursing and Health Care Economics. Districts were consolidated into eight regional Chapters.

As the Detroit District was combined with other districts to become the SE Michigan Chapter, the district donated money for nurse artwork to be placed in the MNA headquarters in Okemos – artist Carol Guskey's four watercolor paintings depict nursing in a clinic examination room, a home care setting, a teaching environment and in an emergency room.

MNA leadership transitioned as Carol Franck retired at the end of 1999 after 13 years as Executive Director. The Carol E. Franck Leadership Award was created in her name.

Nurses in Action

In addition to the three watercolors shown below, a fourth painting by Carol Guskey,
picturing a clinic examination room, is also displayed at MNA headquarters.

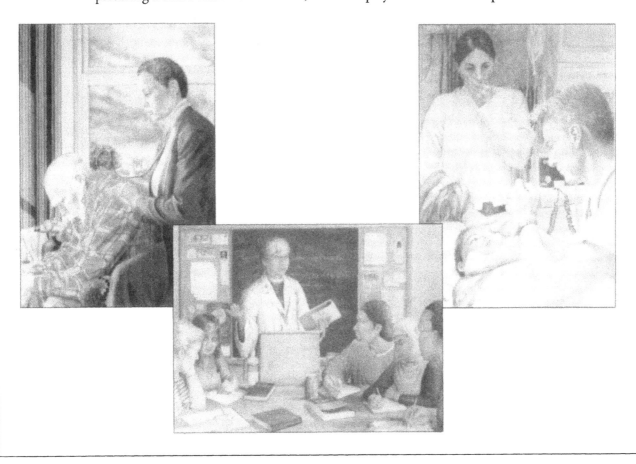

As 2000 approached, MNA leadership worked together to create a vision for the future through a Strategic Plan which included three major goals. While some of the language used might have differed from 1904, the original direction and passion of the organization remains the same:

- Promote quality health care by protecting and enhancing professional nursing practice;

- Advance economic and professional security for registered nurses; and

- Provide programs and services that ensure viability of the Association.

Membership categories were also expanded to include Life Members – RNs who have been MNA members for 30 years or more. Student membership was expanded to include a NexGen category which allowed nursing students to join MNA with limited membership benefits.

An additional 7,500 square feet was added to MNA headquarters in Okemos in 2000, expanding office, storage and meeting room space. The meeting room wing was funded with a bequest from former MNA board member Helen Perrott. And MNA opened the Marquette office in Michigan's Upper Peninsula in June of 1994. At the time, there were approximately 875 nurses at 13 facilities in the Upper Peninsula.

The Michigan Nurses Foundation (MNF) was also created in 2000. The Foundation provides scholarships to nursing students who are entering the workforce, as well as nurses who are continuing their education; awards research grants to researchers exploring "best practices" or addressing critical workplace practice issues; and gives financial aid to nurses who are impaired by chemical dependency and are attending a qualified treatment program, thus assisting them to re-enter the workforce. MNF is a not-for-profit organization funded by individual contributions.

As the use of home computers grew among nurses, technology changed the way MNA members communicated with each other, and how information was made available to members, the nursing community, and health care consumers. A 1996 survey of MNA members revealed only 2% had email address, and the question of creating an MNA website was raised. Three years later MNA launched www.minurses.org. The following year, members could choose, for the first time, to receive MNA's weekly news publication, *Nurseline*, by email. The paper version of *NurseLine* was eliminated in 2003, as the majority of MNA leadership had adopted electronic communication as the preferred method of delivery. The use of technology transformed the work of the Association in other ways, as phone conferences and electronic mailing of documents, reduced costs and increased information transfer.

Nursing education and continuing education were also transformed as geographic constraints were eliminated. Technology, coupled with the implementation of mandatory continuing education rules for nurses in Michigan effective April 1, 1997, revolutionized education. "On-line" distance learning programs became the norm. In response, MNA offered a series of "self-study continuing education models," available first by mail, then electronically through the MNA website site, www.minurses.org.

The words "nursing shortage" became more frequent (again) in 2000. Dr. Peter Buerhaus, Associate Dean for Research, Professor and Valere Potter Distinguished Chair at Vanderbilt University School of Nursing, was the keynote speaker at convention, and presented current data and projections for an impending nursing crisis in the year 2010, as the bulk of nurses retire just when their baby boomer peers will demand more health care. The nursing community across the state banded together to respond. MNA launched a campaign to attract more nurses into the profession. Recruitment materials, including brochures, posters and a video were created and distributed across the state.

In 2001, the Michigan Health and Safety Coalition Nursing Staffing Task Force, which had strong MNA member involvement, looked at the impending and current nursing shortage, and identified the impact nursing care has on "patient safety and health outcomes." One result was creation of a Michigan Center for Nursing, operated by the Michigan Health Council with grant funding from the Michigan Department of Consumer and Industry Services.

These efforts, combined with a downturn in the Michigan economy, turned around the declining nursing school enrollment trend. The result is that today, nursing schools, which were already looking for faculty and facing a huge wave of retirements, are struggling to find faculty and clinical space to meet the burgeoning demand.

A shortage of nurses, difficult working conditions, conflicting viewpoints among nurses, and an ever-changing practice environment are the reality of 2004, as MNA enters the second century of nursing's voice in Michigan. However, the lesson learned from the first hundred years is this: despite the obstacles, internal and external, the registered nurses of Michigan always find a way to carry on!

2004 forward

by Carol Feuss and Lisa Gottlieb-Kinnaird

Timeline

October, 2003 – MNA's Centennial
Celebration kicks off during the
annual convention

May 5, 2004 – A Centennial Gala
celebrates 100 years of Michigan
nursing

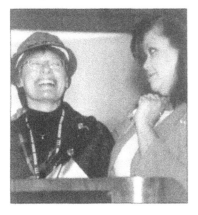

*Outgoing President Marylee
Pakieser, RN, (l) received a special
decorated hat from Southwestern
chapter President Pam Chapman,
RN (r).*

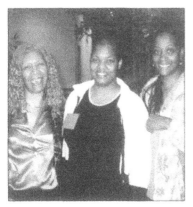

*Student nurses share happy smiles
as they participate in Convention
activities.*

MNA Launches a Year-Long Celebration of Nurses and Nursing

While looking forward to the next century, MNA members and friends took time to celebrate the first 100 years as Michigan's voice for nursing. The Centennial Kickoff took place during the 2003 Convention at the Kalamazoo Radisson Hotel.

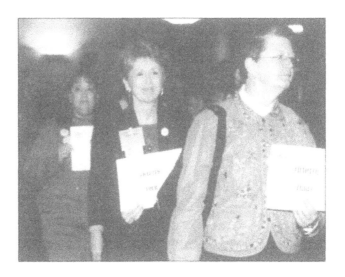

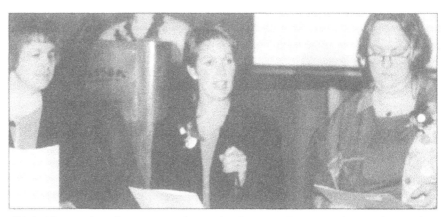

(Top) Chapter Presidents processed into the Opening Ceremony. (Bottom) Members of the Southwestern Chapter (5) performed a moving reading about the diversity of nursing, written by Pat Underwood, RN, PhD (excerpted text on page 108).

Can you help?

I am a new graduate. I can make a difference by bringing fresh enthusiasm and energy to the workplace. I can look with new eyes at what we are doing as we try to provide quality care for all our patients. It is important to me that experienced and expert nurses help me understand why doing things in a certain way will be more effective.

Can you help?

I am an expert medical-surgical nurse. I love giving care at the bedside. I can make a difference by welcoming and mentoring new graduates. I will encourage them to stay at the bedside, so there will be expert nurses to take my place when I retire. It is important to me that we give the best care possible to hospitalized patients. We also need to think about the support they and their families will need after they are discharged. I have an 80 year old patient who is scheduled for discharge after a hip replacement. We have given her lots of individualized teaching and support, but she is not ready to go back to her apartment. Her family is too far away to have her live with them.

Can you help?

I am a rehab nurse practicing in a nursing home. I can make a difference by helping this lady to return to maximum independence. I will assist in mobilizing the support of her family and friends. This is critical in achieving the positive attitude that will speed her recovery. It is important to me . . .

And so the reading went as the Chapter 5 members stood together in a line that stretched beyond the length of the stage. Each nurse linked directly to their area of practice and shared proudly their role in nursing, ending with a poignant question to first the nurse next to them, then to the audience: **Can you help?**

Participants in the reading, written by Patricia Underwood, RN, PhD, were: Kathy Sharp Rosema, RN, BSN; Becky Baldwin, RN; Dee Dray, RN; Jackie Wylie, RN, MSN; Sharon Western, RN; Pat Meave, RN; Andrea Bostrom, RN, PhD; Nate Hoffman, RN; Linda Scott, RN, PhD; Maggie Guthaus, RN, MSN; and Helen Truss, RN, MA.

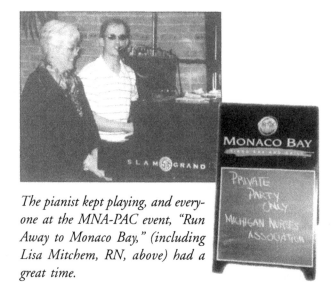

The pianist kept playing, and everyone at the MNA-PAC event, "Run Away to Monaco Bay," (including Lisa Mitchem, RN, above) had a great time.

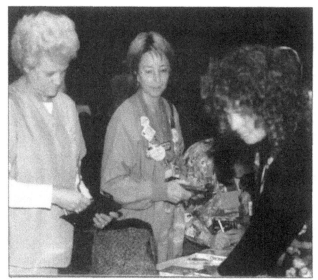

The music of labor singer Anne Feeney was very popular, and participants lined up to purchase her CDs.

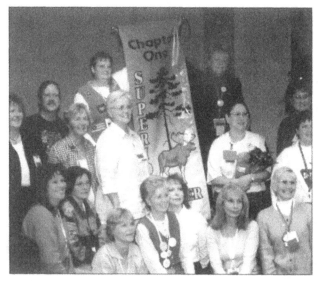

Superior Chapter (1) displayed nursing pride, with a banner created especially for the occasion.

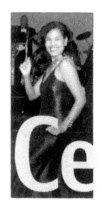

☆ ☆ ☆ ☆ ☆ ☆ *Gala!*

T ributes and reminiscences kicked off MNA's Centennial Gala on May 7, 2004. Held at the Sheraton Lansing Hotel, the evening celebrated "The Legacy of Michigan Nursing". The black-tie-optional event brought nurses and friends of nursing from across the state for an evening of celebration. TV-6 WLNS anchorwoman Sherry Jones emceed the event. Greetings were brought by Marty Gibbs on behalf of Governor Jennifer Granholm; Lansing Mayor Tony Benavides; and Rita Munley Gallagher, RN, PhD, on behalf of the American Nurses Association. But the main focus was celebrating – the past, the present, and the future.

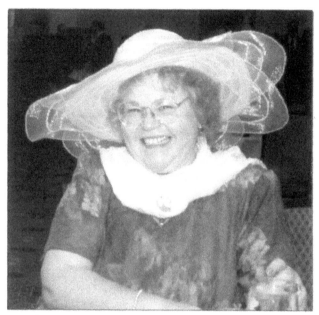

100th Anniversary Steering Committee Co-Chair Mona White, RN, enjoys the night of celebration in her party hat.

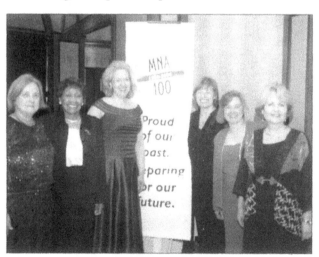

Six MNA presidents attended the Centennial Gala (l-r) Linda Mondoux (1993-1997), Regina Williams (1983-1985), Kimberly Hickey (1997-1999), Marylee Pakieser (1999-2003, Cheryl Johnson (2003-2005) and Patricia Underwood (1989-1993). (Not pictured from this era is Joann Wilcox, 1985-1989). Under their direction, the Michigan Nurses Association became a powerful voice for nursing as the world moved into the 21st century. We honor their leadership which shaped the past and set the vision for the future.

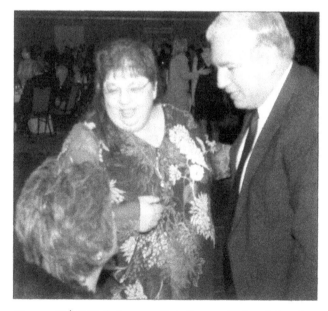

Former E&GW chairperson Jody Berney, RN and Associate Executive Director of Labor Relations John Karebian chat with John's wife, Terri (foreground).

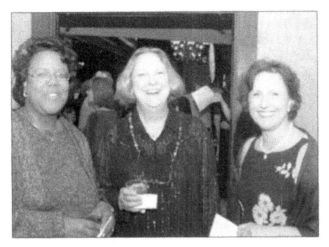

Linda Scott, RN, Andrea Bostrom, RN, and former MNA Director of Government Affairs Judy Pendergast, RN, renew old friendships.

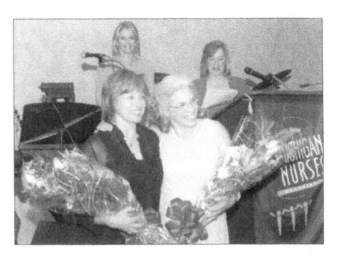

MNA President Cheryl Johnson, RN, thanks Gala Co-Chairs Marylee Pakieser, RN and Victoria Boyce, RN for making the evening a success. In the background is emcee Sherry Jones, TV-6 anchorwoman.

STATE OF MICHIGAN
OFFICE OF THE GOVERNOR
LANSING

JENNIFER M. GRANHOLM
GOVERNOR

JOHN D. CHERRY, JR.
LT. GOVERNOR

May 7, 2004

Dear Friends:

It is an honor and privilege to offer my heartfelt greetings and highest congratulations to the Michigan Nurses Association on its 100th Anniversary.

I commend each member of the Michigan Nurses Association for your commitment to quality healthcare across the state. Let me be among the first to thank you for giving so selflessly to your fellow citizens throughout the past 100 years through quality healthcare services. You have truly made a difference in your communities.

Again, congratulations on your historic 100th Anniversary. Thank you for your contributions to your local community and the state of Michigan.

Sincerely,

Jennifer M. Granholm
Governor

110

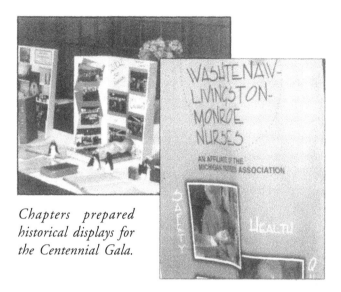

Chapters prepared historical displays for the Centennial Gala.

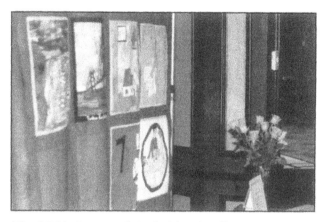

The MNA Centennial Quilt (above) will contain a square from each of MNA's eight chapters. The completed quilt will be displayed at MNA headquarters.

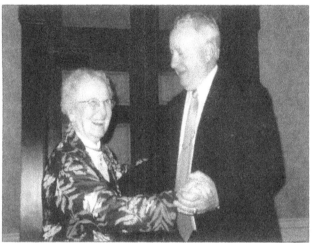

93 years young, Gertrude Stapish, RN, the oldest nurse present, enjoys a dance with her son, Edward Stapish, Jr.

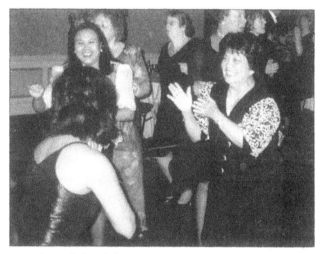

Members of the Philippine Nurses Association of Michigan (PNAM) came to help us celebrate, and we were delighted to have them.

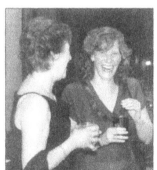

(Left) Julia Stocker, RN (r) shares a laugh with Mary Killeen, RN (l).

(Below l) Dorothy Coye, RN, (l) and her niece, Jan Coye, RN, (r) are former MNA staff members.

(Below r) Nettie Riddick, RN, and Lionel Doyle enjoy the evening.

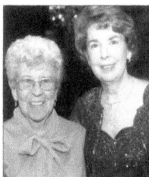

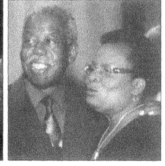

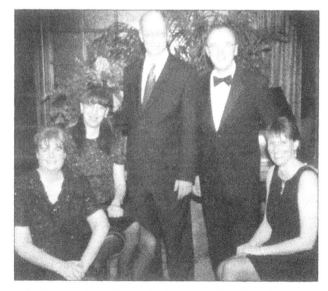

The Centennial History Book team enjoy the celebration. (L-r) Ann Sincox, Lisa Gottlieb-Kinnaird, Tom Bissonnette, Jess Merrill, and Carol Feuss.

Appendices

MNA Presidents Through the Century

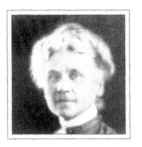

Lystra Gretter
1904-1905

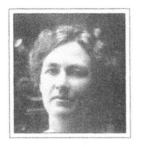

Anna Barbara Switzer
1909-1910

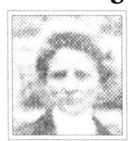

Susan Fisher Apted
1910-1912

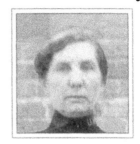

Fantine Pemberton
1912-1914

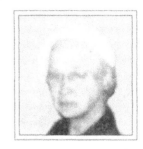

Marion Parks Morse
1919-1921

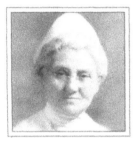

Mary A. Welsh
1923-1926

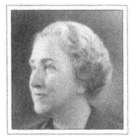

Grace Ross
1926-1928

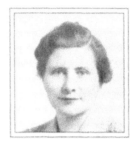

Emilie Sargent
1928-1932

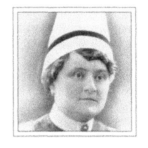

Amy Beers
1932-1933

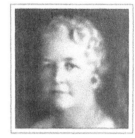

Ann Hellner
1933-1934

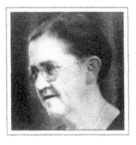

Elba Morse
1934-1936

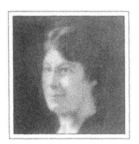

Marion Durrell
1936-1938

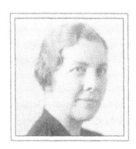

Mabel McNeel
1938-1940

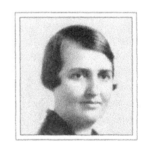

Louise Knapp
1940-1941

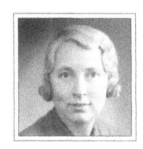

M. Annie Leitch
1941-1942

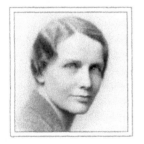

Ella McNeil
1942-1944

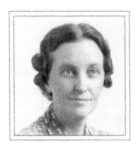

Thelma Brewington
1944-1945

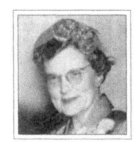

Winifred Kellogg
1945-1946

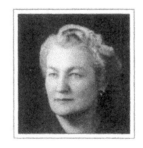

Kathleen F. Sands Young
1946-1947

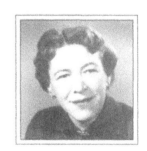

Elizabeth Hilborn
1947-1948

Not pictured: Sarah Sly, 1905-1907; Elizabeth Parker, 1907-1909; Ida M. Barrett, 1914-1917; Elizabeth Parker, 1917-1919; Barbara Bartlett, 1921-1923

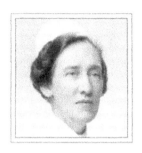

Elizabeth S. Moran
1948-1949

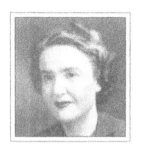

Rhoda Reddig Russell
1949-1950

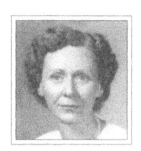

Mildred McFerren
1950-1952

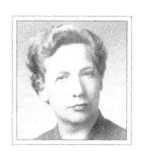

Emma Antcliff
1952-1953

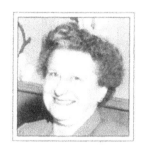

Florence Kempf
1953-1955

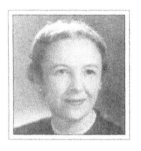

Phyllis MacKay
1955-1959

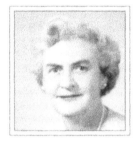

Patricia Walsh
1959-1961

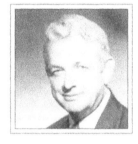

Luther Christman
1961-1965

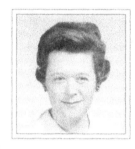

Jessie V. Pergrin
1965-1967

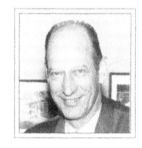

John Wick
1967-1971

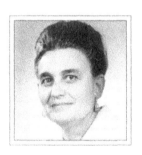

Barbara Horn
1971-1975

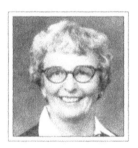

Ann Zuzich
1975-1979

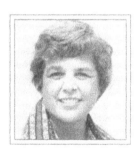

Dorothea Milbrandt
1979-1983

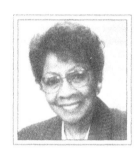

Regina Williams
1983-1985

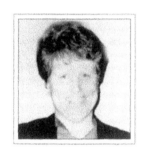

Joann Wilcox
1985-1989

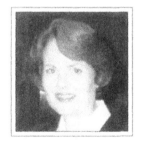

Patricia Underwood
1989-1993

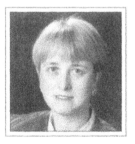

Linda Mondoux
1993-1997

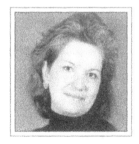

Kimberly Hickey
1997-1999

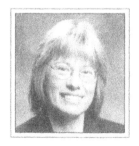

Marylee Pakieser
1999-2003

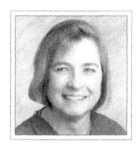

Cheryl Johnson
2003-present

Not pictured: Margaret Shetland, 1950-1950.

Executive Directors Through the Century

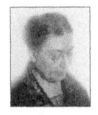
Mary Curtis Wheeler
1925-1929

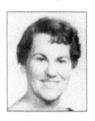
Eleanor M. Tromp Verlee
1961-1968

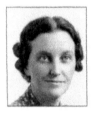
Olive Sewell
1930-1944

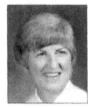
Joan S. Guy
1968-1979

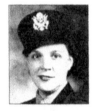
Thelma Brewington
1944-1946

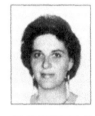
Nadine M. Furlong
1979-1985

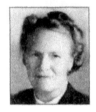
Martha McCrary
1946

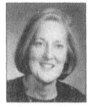
Carol E. Franck
1986-1999

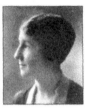
Hulda Edman
1946-1950

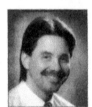
Thomas W. Renkes
1999-2002

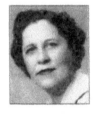
Jean Truckey
1950-1953

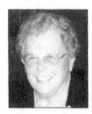
Dorothea M. Milbrandt
2002-2003

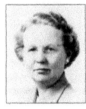
Hazel E. Gabrielson
1953-1960

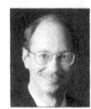
Thomas Bissonnette
2003-present

NOTE: The title of the staff person responsible for the Michigan (State) Nurses Association was "Executive Secretary" until 1952. In that year, the title changed to "Executive Director."

Board of Directors 2004

Cheryl Johnson, President

Julia Stocker, Vice President

Carolyn Hietamaki, Secretary

Diane Goddeeris, Treasurer

Becky Baldwin, Economic & General Welfare Representative

Janet Bodell, Congress on Nursing Practice Representative

Kimberly Ford, Chapter 6 Representative

Gail Jehl, Economic & General Welfare Representative

Lola Johnson, Congress on Nursing & Health Care Economics Representative

Mary Killeen, Chapter 7 Representative

Sue Meeker, Congress on Public Policy Representative

Sandra Merkel, Chapter 8 Representative

Kristine Michaelson, Chapter 1 Representative

Kathryn Oppenheim, Economic & General Welfare Representative

Helen Roznowski, Chapter 2 Representative

Lisa Sylvest, Economic & General Welfare Representative

Helen Truss, Chapter 5 Representative

Vacant, Chapter 3 Representative

Vacant, Chapter 4 Representative

Vacant, Congress on Public Policy Representative

MNA Economic & General Welfare Cabinet 2004

Carolyn Hietamaki, President

John Armelagos, Vice President & Liaison to Michigan AFL-CIO

Elizabeth O'Connor-Rogers, Secretary/Treasurer

Mark Carlson

Romayne Dray

Robert Ehnis

Kimberly Ford

Patricia Meave

Donna Nussdorfer

Kathryn Oppenheim

Chapter Presidents 2004

Kristine Michaelson, Chapter 1

Myrna Holland, Chapter 2

Susan Fogarty, Chapter 3

Sandra Smith, Chapter 4

Becky Baldwin, Chapter 5

Gail Grannell, Chapter 6

Linda Taft, Chapter 7

Opal Lesse, Chapter 8

CYNTHIA B. AGLE, RN, born Dec. 18, 1945, Detroit, MI. Assignments: St. Mary's Hospital, Saginaw, MI, ICU asst./CCU charge; Lapeer County General Hospital, day charge; Mid-Michigan Regional Medical Center, Clare, MI, prevention educator.

Education: St. Mary's Alumni member (graduated with honors); RN, BS, University of Michigan Health Care and Human Behavior; Diploma, BS University of Michigan (graduated with honors), certified hyprotherapy prevention ICRC.

Professional Activities: MNA new graduate board member, FACE Truth and Clarity on Alcohol, board member and past chair of American Cancer Society for state of Michigan.

She worked in Gladwin County teaching substance abuse prevention education with the Duncan Series, 1987-97, wrote curriculum. Today she is executive director of the Michigan Resource Center, a part of the Traffic Safety Association of Michigan, a state clearing nurse for ATOD and Traffic Safety Education material. Cynthia is widowed and has one son.

PAULA J. ALTENBURG, RN, ADN, Staff Nurse, born Aug. 2, 1964, Canton, IL. Education: LPN Certificate, Bay de Noc, Escanaba; RN, Bay de Noc, Escanaba; working on BSN through LSSU. She is listed in *Who's Who of Occupational Health Nurses,* 2000-01.

Assignments: Blue Lake Fine Arts Camp, Muskegon, MI; camp nurse, Group Work Camp, North Dakota; mission nurse, STORA ENSO, Niagara, WI; occupational health nurse, Dickinson County Health Care System; RN, Emergency, Iron Mountain, MI.

Activities: CPR instructor, PALS, ACLS, TNCC, breath alcohol tech and hearing conservationist.

Accomplishments: Going back to school full-time and having a husband, Neal William Altanburg Jr., and three children: Diana, Michelle and William; graduating with LPN certificate and working full time as LPN while going to school full time for RN.

Paula is now working part time as RN in emergency dept. DCHS in Iron Mountain, MI and going to school part time for BSN.

ANN KATHRYN ANGUS, RN, Staff Nurse, born Nov. 11, 1945 in Rochester, MI. Education: Honor Society in high school/top 10; voted most athletic in high school; foreign exchange student; captain of volley ball, baseball and basketball, HS; treasurer HS class for two years; played college basketball and was also captain.

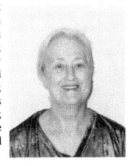

Awards/Honors: received Good Citizen Award, Professional Business Women's Scholarship Award; associate degree in nursing, Oakland Community College. Ann was elected MNA convention representative, two terms, union representative and six years for Staff RNs at LRH.

Assignments include OR, Scrub RN and Circulator, William Beaumont Royal Oak; Pontiac Osteopathic; Wheelock Hospital, Goodrich, MI, OR Scrub/Circulator ER Staff; ER Staff RN and now PACU RN at Lapeer Regional Hospital.

She is president of her own corporation as a real estate investor; director of Adoration at Catholic Church for 12 years; Girl Scout leader for four years; 4-H leader for seven years in sewing, horses, public speaking, writing, stain glass and photography.

Married 33 years to Richard Angus and they have two daughters, Kate and Sara, and are helping rear 2-year-old grandson and infant granddaughter. Kate is an elementary teacher and Sara at OCC in CAD Program.

BIRTHALE ARCHIE, RN, born in Houston, MS and became interested in health care when she was only 13 years old. She decided to become an RN when a nurse recruiter spoke to her school about a two-year RN program.

She was one of an initial class of 32 with only 16 graduating. She received an associate degree in applied arts and science and obtained her license to practice as an RN.

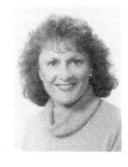

She received the MNA Bertha Lee Culp Human Rights Award in 2002, National Black Nurses Association RN Community Service Award for 2002 and many other honors.

She is a member of the Board of Directors of the MNA representing the Lakeshore Chapter, member of Michigan Nurses Foundation, lifetime member of NBNA and founder and president of the West Michigan Regional Kalamazoo-Muskegon, MI Chapter of NBNA.

She obtained a BS in biology and chemistry from Aquinas College in 1978 and her MSN from Wayne State University in 1986.

She is a member of First Community AME Church in Grand Rapids, and is a child of God leaning on His Grace and understanding. She was married and had one son she loved dearly who passed away in 1997. She is the founder and CEO for Nursing Care Professionals.

NANCY T. ARTINIAN, PhD, RN, BC, FAHA, is a Professor (promoted in April 2004) and Director of the Doctoral and Postdoctoral Programs in the College of Nursing at Wayne State University. She received her doctoral degree in nursing from Wayne State University in 1988 and completed postdoctoral training in nursing and health promotion/risk reduction at the University of Michigan School of Nursing in 1997.

Dr. Artinian holds certification from the American Nurses Credentialing Center in cardiovascular nursing and is a Fellow of the Council on Cardiovascular Nursing, American Heart Association. She has more than 40 publications and has conducted several funded research studies. Dr. Artinian is currently conducting a study, which is funded by the National Institutes of Health/National Institute of Nursing Research, to test the effects of a home blood pressure telemonitoring intervention on blood pressure control.

FAYE ATANASOFF, RN, BSN, born May 8, 1957 in Stambaugh, MI. Education: BSN, BS in psychology and MBA, all at Northern Michigan University.

Assignments include Float, IMC, Marquette General Hospital; Float, Sparrow, Lansing General Hospital; all areas, charge, diabetes educator, Iron County Community Hospital. Currently working in Outpatient Diabetes Management on an on-call basis about seven hours a week.

Faye researched the feasibility to open home health unit at hospital. Her husband Donn is an attorney and they have three children: Alex, Aubrey and Austin.

ANDRES E. AYALA, RN, born May 8, 1980 in Bogota, Colombia. Graduated in Spring 2003 from Oakland Community College and is now working in Medical Critical Care ICU at Henry Ford Hospital. She is married to Paola Ayala.

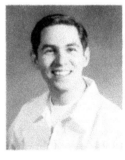

FLO BAERREN, Labor Relations Representative, Flo joined the MNA staff in the summer of 1998. She represents several staff councils. Flo is involved in all aspects of collective bargaining, including contract negotiation, grievance resolution, training, and arbitration preparation.

She came to the MNA after working for the Michigan Court of Appeals as a public information representative. Her background also includes processing unemployment compensation claims and experience as a litigation legal assistant at a private law firm.

Flo holds a bachelor of arts degree in history from Case-Western Reserve University and a master's in labor relations and human resources from Michigan State University's School of Labor and Industrial Relations. She also earned a certificate as a legal assistant from Lansing Community College.

Memorable experience was when a legal assistant with Jackson County prosecutor and she researched a criminal issue which was eventually argued at U.S. Supreme Court and established the law on this issue.

Flo has two sons, Al and Eric, daughter Jennifer, and grandson Sam.

NANCY (CHAMPAGNE) BAILEY,

became interested in nursing as a pre-teen in Flint, MI while hospitalized with a severe leg infection. After marriage and three children, she became a RN in 1976 obtaining her ADN from Mott Community College.

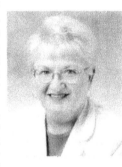

In 1987, working as a critical care nurse at St. Joseph's Hospital in Flint, she completed her BSN from the University of Michigan. She was a clinical instructor at the Hurley School of Nursing about a year before accepting a position as a Critical Care Nurse Educator at St. Joseph's. She held that position until obtaining her MSN from Saginaw Valley State University in 2000. She currently is a cardiology clinical nurse specialist at Genesys Regional Medical Center.

She is a member of the ANA, MNA Bay-Central Chapter, American Association of Critical Care Nurses and Sigma Theta Tau. She volunteers at the Flint Free Clinic, Crim. Medical tent and Habitat for Humanity. She also teaches BLS and ACLS.

MARY BAKER, born in Lawrenceville,

IL, her father a physician and mother a nurse. She graduated from St. Olaf College, 1971, BSN, Mankato State University, 1983, MS, and Northern Michigan University, 1997, MSN.

She worked at the Mayo Clinic, Hemodialysis, 1971-77, and Head of Nephrology in Battle Creek, 1978-84. In 1984 she moved to the

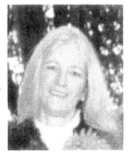

UP working with senior citizens and in a Nursing Center.

She was president of the American Nephrology Nurses Association, 1983-84. Memberships include Sigma Theta Tau, and past board member for UP HIV/AIDS RCPG. She has presented in Italy and Spain.

Her involvement with MNA has been Ethics, Nominating, Membership/Marketing Committees, the PAC Board and the Great Lakes Chapter.

She was president of Les Cheneaux Islands Association and chairperson of Clark Township Planning Commission.

She loves to garden, cook and attend cooking classes. She is married to a radiologist with similar interests and love for their toy poodles.

CYNTHIA A. BEEL-BATES, Dr., Re-

search Associate II, Lecturer, born May 22, 1952, Mt. Clemens, MI. She read Cherry Ames books as a child and read a *Reader's Digest* condensed book about ship *Hope*. By 5th grade she decided to be a nurse and never once wavered. She considered it her vocation and wishes to thank Dr. Donna Algase for her mentorship.

She received her BSN from Nazareth College, MI; MSN from Wayne State University; certificate in aging and PhD from University of Michigan.

Cynthia worked 13 months ICU at Bongess; three years at Kalamazoo County Health Dept.; six years at St. Joseph Mercy Hospital as Gerontological Clinical Nurse Specialist; two years at Botsford, continuing care; 14 years at UM School of Nursing where she is currently doing research and teaching. Also, teaches at Madonna University and GVSU and clinical at Huron Woods.

In 1988 she received Outstanding Gerontological Nurse of the Year. Professional activities include Sigma Theta Tau, Gerontological Society of America, National Association of Clinical Nurse Specialists.

Accomplishments include MNA/ANA delegate; chairperson, Congress on Public Policy, 2003-04; Hartford Foundation Summer Fellow, 2003.

Married to David for 24 years, they have daughter Meredith and son Michael.

NATHALIE WALKER BEARD, born

in Grenada, MS, was encouraged to become a registered nurse by Louise Reed, a Jamaican missionary RN. Nathalie's professional journey includes staff nurse at Harper Hospital and Detroit General Hospital, community health nurse at Wayne State Uni-

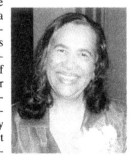

versity Health Care Institute, executive director of the Detroit American Indian Health Center and nurse consultant survey monitor and licensing officer for the Michigan Department of Public Health.

She was 1982-83 vice chair of the MNA Human Rights Commission, 1989-90 program director of Detroit District MNA and MNA's 1990 Staff Nurse of the Year award.

Nathalie received her ADDN from Wayne County Community College and her BSN and MSN from Wayne State University.

Her 1983 *"Your Diabetes Book"* was funded by the Chronic Disease Control Division, Michigan Department of Public Health. She is currently writing a book on Detroit's historical North End.

She is married to Theodore R. Beard Jr.

SHIRLEY DISHAW BECK, Critical

Care Staff Nurse, Pulmonary Resource Nurse, born June 6, 1960, Iron Mountain, MI. She received her BSN from Northern Michigan University in 1982.

Shirley worked at University Hospital, Madison, WI, 1982-89, and at Dickinson County Healthcare System 1989 to present.

Recipient of Nurse Excellence awards and certified in critical care nursing since 1986, she is active with MNA Chapter I Nominating Committee; DCH Staff Council Board Member and Negotiating Team; MNA State Delegate (seven years); School Health Presentations; and DCH Professional Nurse Practice Committee.

She is married with four children.

JODY BETH BERNEY, Clinical Nurse

Supervisor, Child/Adolescent Psychiatry, born Oct. 9, 1952 in Newark, NJ. Received her BSN in 1974 from University of Michigan.

Assignments with University of Michigan Health System include several roles: staff nurse, clinical care coordinator and currently clinical nurse supervisor, child/adolescent psychiatry.

Awards include 1986 MNA E&GW Achievement Award; 1987 University of Michigan Excellence in Psychiatric Nursing Award; 1994 and 1998 MNA Recognition of Service Award; and 1999 Washlenaw-Livingston Monroe Chapter Nurses Association Nurse of the Year.

She's member of Sigma Theta Tau and has held the past MNA offices of MNA Vice President, 1994-98; Board of Directors, 1990-98; E&GW Cabinet 1986-92, chair, 1990-92; past chair, bylaws; past chair Strategic Plan Committee; ANA Delegate; MNA Delegate; UMPNC past grievance representative and negotiating team member; and ANA Task Force on implementation of ANA staffing guidelines.

Jody's son Daniel James was born Nov. 17, 1992.

JOAN T. BICKES, MSN, APRN, BC, Assistant Professor (Clinical), It was the best decision of her life-to become a nurse! She came from a long line of nurses. Her mother and aunt were nurses. Two sisters and multiple cousins are nurses. She went to college in 1969. She never entertained the idea of becoming a nurse. She wanted to see the world and become an ambassador and live in some exotic part of the world.

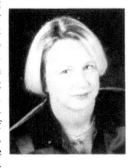

She received her first degree in French and history in December 1972. She went to Europe for six months and decided that she really had to know someone important to become an ambassador. She came back to the U.S. and decided that she needed a job! She had no money. The teaching jobs for language teachers were nil. This is when she began to think that maybe she could be a nurse. Her mother and sisters seemed to like nursing. She applied to Mercy College of Detroit and began taking the required science courses. She had not taken sciences in her previous degree. Then she had to be accepted into the nursing program. At that time MCD took their allotted number of students into the nursing program in the freshman year. She could only get a spot in the class, if someone dropped out. She began looking into diploma and ADN programs because she figured that she already had one degree. Someone was looking out for her because she did get a place in the nursing class in the fall of 1974. This was the second best decision that she made, to get the BSN! She graduated in May 1977 with her BSN.

She worked for a year rotating days and midnights at Children's Hospital of Michigan. She worked on the preemie-newborn unit, a step-down unit from the NICU. It was a great experience but she had decided before she left UDM that she wanted to be a Community Health Nurse. She took a position at Oakland County Health Department in August 1978. She was a field nurse in Troy, MI. She made home visits and had five elementary schools, one junior high and one high school as part of her caseload. She loved every minute of the experience.

After a year in this position she applied to graduate school at Wayne State University. She had decided she would go to graduate school part-time. However, she received a professional traineeship and had to give up her full-time job to attend school full-time. Another big decision had to be made.

Her third best career decision was to attend graduate school full-time! She continued to work at the health department as a part-time clinic nurse, which gave her some new and different skills. In May 1981 she graduated with her MSN in community health nursing and a minor in education. She continued to work part-time through the next 12 years with many varied experiences.

She worked as a clinical instructor at WSU, OU and UM. She was a research assistant doing a hypertension intervention study at the Detroit Health Department and she was a research assistant at Beaumont Hospital doing nursing intervention with radiation oncology patients. All of these experiences helped her grow as a nursing professional.

At the same time she was an active member of the MNA, ANA, and her local district.

She was inducted into Sigma Theta Tau. She has also received the Leadership award from the Michigan Public Health Association.

In 1993 she became a full-time instructor at Wayne State University. She became certified in CHN in 2001. She is now an assistant professor (clinical). She remains active in professional organizations. She seeks out new opportunities for her students.

She hopes to take a group of nursing students from WSU for an alternative experience to India next spring. She feels like she has become an ambassador for nursing.

She has enjoyed her journey in nursing to this point and looks forward to many more years in this challenging and worthwhile profession.

KATHLEEN BIRDSALL, born Kathleen Donohoe, in Detroit, MI, became interested in nursing after being a wife and mother of two little girls. A surgical experience, in which a registered nurse made a profound impact on her, convinced Kathleen this was the career/calling for which she had been searching.

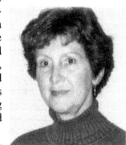

She graduated at age 32 from Henry Ford Community College's Dearborn, MI, ADN, program, received her BSN Ferris State University 15 years later. Her chosen field has been cardiology nursing for all of her career, beginning in the critical care setting, and currently in cardiac rehabilitation. She is certified by the ANCC in cardiac rehabilitation and by the American College of Sports Medicine as an exercise specialist.

She has been an active member of MNA since 1993, serving on the Congress for Public Policy and the Congress for Nursing and Health Care Economics. She has learned much about the workings of a large member association as an elected delegate to state and national conventions.

Her special interests are world travel with her husband of 37 years and two daughters, scuba diving, and hiking. She has a love of animals, especially dogs, and she is a passionate pacifist and public speaker on active lifestyle.

THOMAS "TOM" BISSONNETTE, MS, RN, was born and reared in Bay City, MI. He is the fourth of Gerald and Viola (Hart) Bissonnette's eight children. Tom has many nurses in his family tree, including his paternal grandmother, an aunt, his mother who graduated from the Mercy School of Nursing in Grand Rapids, and two sisters who graduated from the Delta College School of Nursing in Bay City.

Tom entered the Navy upon his high school graduation and became a hospital corpsman, serving in Chicago and Boston. At Naval Hospital Boston, he was influenced by several Navy nurses, including Joan Bartik, Janice (Long) Johnson, and Kate Krumm. Following his active duty in the Navy he entered the University of Michigan School of Nursing while participating in the Naval Reserves. Prior to his sophomore year of college, Tom married Molly Benner, whom he had met during their junior year of high school together.

During his junior and senior years of college, Tom worked as a nursing assistant on 6-West of the old Main Hospital at U of M, where he was influenced by several of his nurse co-workers, though most importantly by Annie Withers. He was elected the senior class president of U of M's Nursing School Class of 1979. Molly and Tom's 10-day-old daughter Anne attended his college convocation.

Upon graduation from U of M, Tom worked in psychiatric nursing at the University of Michigan Hospitals as a staff nurse, clinical nurse educator, and as an assistant head nurse. While working on the Clinical Studies Unit, affectionately known as NPI-6, Betty Kelsch, Linda (Melman) Powell, and Nancy Barber were nurse leaders who were role models for him. Tom also was a member of the U of M Professional Nurse Council negotiation team in 1981 and 1983. Margo Barron, Jody Berney, and Debbie Hartwick mentored him in how best to advocate for staff nurses within collective bargaining during this time.

Tom returned to school to earn his master's of science degree in psychiatric nursing from the U of M in 1984, with a specialist in aging certificate from the Institute of Gerontology. Tom and Molly's five-year-old daughter Anne and two-year-old daughter Theresa helped to celebrate this graduation. Faculty important to Tom's growth during his undergraduate and graduate studies included Janice Lindberg, Arlene Hegedus, Reg Williams, and Bonnie Hagerty.

In 1985, Tom accepted the position of clinical nurse manager of St. Joseph Hospital's Mercywood Psychiatric Hospital Older Adult Unit in Ann Arbor. During his 10 years in this position, he participated in a move to a new hospital building, several physical plant and program downsizings, the planning and implementation of a clinical research Alzheimer's unit, contributed to a book on understanding the difficult behaviors of the victims of Alzheimer's disease, and co-led the nurse manager leadership group. Colleagues who supported Tom during these years included Christeen Holdwick, Judy Coucouvanis, Michael Kraft and Mary Olson.

Upon leaving St. Joe's in 1996, Tom worked in a variety of settings, including a quality management and a geriatric case management company. He also worked as a geropsychiatric clinical nurse specialist in long term care settings. Tom started work as a case manager for health care professionals impaired due to substance abuse or mental illness in 1998, eventually becoming the program director for Michigan and Indiana's impaired professionals programs. Nurse colleagues during these years included Tom Renkes and Caryl Prati.

In the fall of 2003, Tom accepted the executive director position for the Michigan Nurses Association. He had been a member of MNA for 25 years, provided leadership as a chapter president and a member of the state Board of Directors, as well as serving as a chapter and state delegate. Tom resides in Ann Arbor with Molly, his wife of 28 years and an assortment of pets.

DEANNA K. BITNER, RN, BSN, Director of Hospice at Great Lakes Home Health

and Hospice in Jackson, MI. She was born Feb. 5, 1962, Port Clinton, OH. She has been a nurse for 20 years, held license in Ohio, New York and Michigan with 10 years management experience.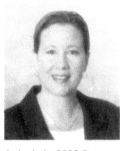

Personal awards include 2002 International Who's Who in Professional Management, 2004 Manchester's Who's Who in Professional Management.

Deanna is a member of Michigan Hospice and Palliative Care Organization, Michigan Hospice and Palliative Nurse Association, MNA and National Female Executive Organization. She sat on the board of directors for Michigan Hospice and Palliative Organization, 2001-02.

She graduated in 1984 with associate degree of applied science in nursing from University of Toledo; graduated magna cum laude from college in 2001 with bachelor's degree in applied science in nursing. Deanna is currently pursuing her master's degree from U of M.

Deanna is married with three children, ages 10, 16 and 17.

JANET BODELL, born in Detroit, discerned a calling to become a registered nurse from an early age. Stories of WWII nurses

and reading books about nurses assisted with her decision. She was a member of the Future Nurses Club at Hazel Park High School.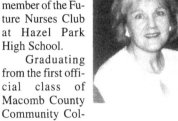

Graduating from the first official class of Macomb County Community College in 1971, she received an associate degree in science-nursing and obtained her license to practice as RN.

After working in Med-Surg at Bi-County Hospital, Janet worked five years in the Recovery Room at Riverside Osteopathic Hospital in Trenton. The last 17 years she has been a nurse administrator at South Shore Ambulatory Center for Surgery.

She earned a BS in professional arts from St. Joseph's College in Maine, 1999; a MS in hospice from Madonna University in 2002; and is currently completing a MS in nursing-education from St. Joseph's College-Maine. She is a published professional author.

She is a Professed Secular Franciscan from St. Bonaventure's Fraternity in Detroit and a member of Our Lady of the Woods Catholic Church. She is married to John E. Bodell, D.O. and has one daughter, Dawn M. Bodell, D.O. who resides in Eugene, OR.

LINDA D. LEE BOND, was born in Missaukee County, MI. A high school teacher, a favorite aunt, and "Cherry Ames" influenced her decision to enter nursing. She started her education at Butterworth Hospital School of Nursing, then stopped to marry her high school sweetheart and have two children.

She completed an ADN at Henry Ford Community College, MSN at Wayne State University and PhD in family ecology from Michigan State University.

Her nursing specialty is obstetrics and family. For many years she practiced at a small community hospital in a variety of roles. An opportunity to teach in a practical nursing program led to a career in nursing education spanning more than 30 years, teaching primarily at the university level.

She has been active in nursing organizations serving at all levels; was an accreditation visitor for NLNAC and a delegate to MNA and ANA; and was honored with the Outstanding Contribution to MNA award in 2002.

KATHERINE BRADLEY, born in Detroit at the former Women's Hospital (Hutzel) and lived in the city for over 25 years. She attended St. Alphonsus, grade school and Immaculate High School, where she was awarded the "Outstanding Student in the

School" during her sophomore year. She earned her BS degree at Mercy College at the suggestion of her family physician who told her that he felt "nurses were going toward earning their degrees in a college 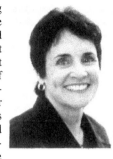 atmosphere." While there, she was president of Theta Alpha Chi nursing sorority. Upon graduation, she began her active duty service in the Navy, graduating "with distinction" from Officer's Indoctrination School.

While rearing five children, she earned MS in nursing degree and her PhD in instructional technology at Wayne State University. She began her teaching career with Oakland Community College, teaching pediatrics during summer sessions. She taught pediatric nursing at Mercy College of Detroit as a full-time instructor and later directed the Extended Campus Program for ADN to BSN completion, retiring from there in 1996 as an associate professor.

Next, Dr. Bradley became program coordinator for nursing at Wayne County Community College, followed by her selection to Director of Nursing. In 1998, she became the Associate Dean of Nursing at Henry Ford Community College and presently retains that position.

Dr. Bradley is a retired captain in the U.S. Navy Nurse Corps, where she spent over 20 years in a variety of command positions, including medical unit training officer, executive officer, nursing school liaison officer and commanding officer. Her last assignment was as commanding officer of a Fleet Hospital Unit. She had four years of active duty split service, 1960-62, and 1992-95 serving in Medical-Surgical, Pediatric, G.I., Dermatology, and Outpatient Clinics and Wards. Her last assignment on active duty was as Head, Reserve Programs Naval Health Sciences Education and Training Command in Bethesda, MD, where she was in charge of 17,000 medical reservists. Katherine was recalled during Desert Storm where she taught CPR to 132 students and wrote immunization and other policies for the Great Lakes Naval Hospital Command. She earned the Navy Commendation Medal, Navy Achievement Medal w/2 Gold Stars, Navy Meritorious Unit Commendation Medal, National Defense Medal w/Bronze Star, Armed Forces Reserve Medal w/M and Silver Hourglass, Navy Rifle Expert Medal and Navy Pistol Expert Medal.

ARLENE BRENNAN, born May 31, 1947, Manistee, MI. RN for 35 years; nurse practitioner for 15 years until 1993; and currently a consultant, Brennan Executive Transition Management in Health-care.

She has been an MNA member since

being in nursing school; was first MNA "Outstanding Nurse in Advanced Practice in 1986; chairperson of MNA Council of Nurses in Advanced Practice, 1980-84; member of MNA Board of Directors, 1984-90; and MNA representative to BCBS MI Board of Directors.

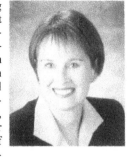

Memorable experience was co-producing breast self-exam video for patients that was distributed nationally.

Earned her ADN at Northwestern MI College; BS at Michigan State University; MSN at Wayne State University and MHSA at University of Michigan.

Married, no children, Arlene is currently health care consulting in the areas of executive transition management and facilitation.

MARGARET PRINCE-BROOKHOUSE,

BSN, RN, is a Bay Central Chapter 4 executive board member and representative to the Congress on Nursing Economics of MNA. She graduated with academic and departmental honors from SVSU in 2003. An active member of SVSU's Student Nurses Association and NSNA, she was recognized for her vision and leadership on the executive board. Margaret also participated in recruitment to nursing through Project Open at SVSU. In 2002 she received an appointment as a Valor nursing student at the Aleda E. Lutz VA Medical Center.

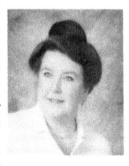

Margaret received an associate in arts from Delta College in 1979 and held various positions in banking, asbestos legal research, retail management, customer sales/service, and was a business owner for 15 years before returning to university.

She previously taught childbirth classes and was a member of Le Leche League. She is a member of the American Society of Pain Management Nurses, Transcultural Nursing Society, MNA and ANA. She is a staff nurse at Covenant Health Care and works per diem at Bay Medical Care Facility.

Margaret is married and the mother of three sons who encouraged her throughout her journey towards nursing.

DEBBIE J. BROWN, RN, BSN, born

Oct. 16, 1956, Bowling Green, OH. In 1979 she earned her RN from Mercy School of Nursing, and in 2001, she returned to school working on BSN completion and finally achieved degree in June 2004 at Eastern Michigan University. It was a struggle but well worth it.

Assignments include 1979-80, Vascular Floor at Mercy Hospital, Toledo, OH; 1980-82, Med/Surg at Mercy Memorial Hospital, Monroe, MI; 1982-97, step-down ICU charge nurse; 1997-present cardiac rehabilitation coordinator at Mercy Memorial Hospital.

Served on Quality Improvement Committee, is ACLS certified and an ACLS instructor. Debbie is currently working in Cardiac Rehab, which is very rewarding.

Married 24 years to Dan, they have three children: Chris (married in summer 2004), Heather and Natalie.

KAREN M. BROWN, RN, MS, went to

the University of Michigan, graduated with a BSN in 1976 and has been an active MNA member since. She was involved in E&GW activities and served as chairperson of Staff Council. Karen returned to U of M to obtain MS in parent-child nursing. As she began teaching and working as a clinical specialist, she was active in Maternal-Child Division and Education Committee. She received the Maternal-Child Health Nurse Achiever Award and chaired the Search/Select Committee for the MNA Executive Director.

Karen began working as a hospital nursing director, and served on the MNA Board representing nursing administration and provided editing for the *Michigan Nurse*. She is dean at Kirtland Community College, including the nursing program. Karen led the development and implementation of an RN from LPN Online Program. She is currently completing a doctoral degree in education leadership.

LORRAINE M. (THOMAS) BROWN,

RN, CNOR, CRNFA, born May 9, 1948, Canton, OH (Stark County). Her assignments include nurse in the OR, June 1969 to September 1969, Canton, OH, Aultman Hospital; September 1969-February 1974, 11-7 charge nurse and 7-3 assistant head nurse; February 1974 to present, OR staff nurse, CNOR, 1980 and CRN first assistant, 1986.

Memorable experiences include attendance at the Association of Peri-Operative Registered Nurses (23) and two world conferences (64).

Lorraine has a diploma and dual certification. She is a graduate of Aultman Hospital School of Nursing. Currently she is completing 30 years at Borgess School of Nursing Medical Center as CRNFA/Service Coordinator for general surgery including OB/GYN Department Based Nursing Practice Committee (two years).

Her mother was RN, Class of 1947 and mother-in-law, RN, Class of 1946, both were graduates of Aultman Hospital School of Nursing. Her father is an electrician. She has two siblings.

DONNA JEAN (FONGER) BUECHE,

AD, BSN, nurse manager for emergency room and Oncology Unit. She was employed at Hurley Medical Center for over 38 years. In 1982 she received the Hurley Medical Center Employee of the Year. She had 14 consecutive years of perfect attendance.

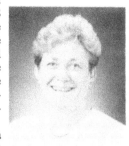

Donna earned her AD at Flint Community Junior College in 1963; BSN at U of M in 1987; and attended Madonna University, 1993. She was born on June 25, 1943 and was admired by all in Owosso, MI. Her positive energy and compassion was an inspiration to all in her presence. She was a nurse and a leader that many students and nurses looked up to, she demonstrated a manner of caring that could only be taught by example. Donna gave the following speech at a nursing graduation ceremony, it contained 10 bits of advice for new graduates to take with them as they ventured out into the real world of nursing.

1) Don't pack away your books, education is ongoing. Don't become stagnant, keep moving, we owe it to our patients and ourselves.

2) Make your practice different from everyone else—be creative. Don't get so caught up in tasks and procedures that you forget to give the personal individual touch to whatever care you give. Patients do not remember the medicine or treatment that was late as much as they remember that the nurse was friendly and kind.

3) Be empathetic—without it, there's no basis for practice.

4) Be unbiased and non-judgmental so everyone feels the same respect.

5) Always remember to be your patient's advocate, because sometimes there isn't anyone else. Virginia Henderson quoted "The nurse is the mouth piece for those too weak and withdrawn to speak."

6) Try to keep a passion about your work. The passion of nursing helps to keep you alive and enthusiastic. Nursing is changing constantly, you need to be flexible and willing to change. I don't believe in burn-out, there are so many options in nursing!

7) Nurses need to be kind to each other. Nurses cannot work alone—we as nurses are each others customers.

8) Keep your sense of humor and light heartedness. There's so much seriousness that we need to keep the right perspective.

9) There is always the challenge of facing the difficult patient or family. I believe in the saying, "Be kind to unkind people, they probably need it the most." People will respond if they know you are sincere.

10) We need to take care of ourselves,

because if we are not healthy, there's nothing left to offer our patients.

Donna closed her speech with a quote from Donna Diers, "Nursing puts us in touch with being human." Nurses are invited into the inner spaces of other people's existence without even asking, for where there is suffering, loneliness, the tolerable pain of cure or the solitary pain of permanent change, there is a need for the kind of human service we call nursing.

Donna passed away in 2002. She is survived by husband Kenneth Beuche, son Ronald and wife Jane Forger, daughter Ronda and husband Andy Little, daughter Kelly and husband Jim Carlson, and four loving grandchildren: Amelia and Shelby Forger and Brett and Courtney Little.

Donna Fonger Beuche was the mother of all nurses. As my mentor I will never forget the impact she had on me as a new grad, manager, colleague, and friend—Diane Welker RN, APRN, BC.

LINDA CANFIELD, born in Alpena, MI, was always interested in helping people, and decided to go into health care at the age of 19.

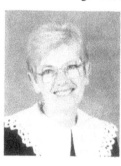

Linda was married with one child at the time. She has worked at Alpena General Hospital for over 30 years starting in June 1971 as a nurses aide. Over the past 32 years Linda was mentored along by her co-workers and supervisors. While she worked she took classes part-time. She earned her LPN, an associate degree in nursing and, finally her BS in nursing.

While working and rearing her family she also was active in the union. First in the United Steel Workers Association who represented the support staff at the hospital, then she held a variety of positions in Alpena MNA staff council. She also served as a delegate many years for MNA and ANA and was a past chair of E&GW. She presently holds a seat on the E&GW Cabinet.

She is married with three children, has six grandchildren and still has a passion for nursing.

CHERYL A. CARLEVATO *see page 165*

PAMELA J. CHAPMAN *see page 165*

MARY CHAROTHRN, born in Keral, South India. She became interested in nursing when she was in high school and went to nursing school in Bombay, India (800 miles from her hometown). Mary received her RN/Midwifery degree in 1969, came to the USA in November 1971, then took her Michigan State Board. She has been working health care

for 32 years and working in ICU for 17 years. Now she is a charge nurse in ICU and also works in ED.

She is a member of MNA and one of the elected officers and negotiating team for their hospital bargaining team. Mary is a chapter treasurer and a previous staff council delegate and MNA delegate.

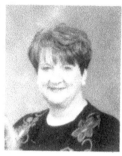

Mary and her husband have been blessed with two beautiful daughters. The oldest is a microbiologist, married, works and lives in Grand Rapids, MI. The younger daughter is going to Western Michigan University studying to be a nurse. Mary is a member of St. Mary's Church in Alpena, MI.

MARY CHERRY, RN, born April 2, 1963, Alpena, MI. She earned her LPN diploma degree at Mercy School of Practical Nursing and RN associate degree, Charles Stewart Mott Community College.

Accomplishments and memorable experiences include ACLS, PALS and TNCC. She is working as RN staff relief for pre-op holding, ER and recovery room.

Mary has been married 19 years and has two children.

LEIGH A. CHILDERS, born April 30, 1955, Flint, MI, has worked in long term care, cardiac home health, in critical care and currently is employed at Lapeer Regional Hospital in the Progressive Care Unit.

With scholarships throughout nursing school, she graduated cum laude from nursing school for both Practical Nursing Certificate and associate degree in applied arts.

Leigh is past president of the local Association for Retarded Citizens; past president of the local Cooperative Nursery School; past secretary, vice president and president of the Lapeer Regional Hospital RN Staff Council; served on the Negotiations Committee with some of the earliest contracts and has worked with many other volunteer groups.

Graduated with honors from St. Clair County Community College in 1992 with associates in applied arts and in 1976 with honors from the same college for LPN certificate. She took a course to become certified in gerontology from the same college in 1978.

Married for 27 years to Charles, she is the mother of two great children: Charles Jr. and Carlee. Carlee is currently attending Mott Community College in Flint and plans to follow in her mother's footsteps by becoming a registered nurse.

Currently, Leigh is attending the University of Phoenix (Flint campus) the pioneering FlexNet course in this area for RN-to-BSN. She plans to graduate in June 2004.

Leigh also enjoys spending time up north at her cottage and playing with her beautiful granddaughter, Sarora.

Leigh decided to become a nurse because of an experience with a long hospitalization at age 17 after a serious car accident. She saw shining examples of angels of mercy and wanted to be a part of a caring profession.

JANE CHRISTNER, born Elkton, MI. Assignments include charge nurse OB/Newborn Nursery; med/surg at Huron Medical Center; school nurse, Laker Schools, 1976-79; H.C.C.M.H., 1981-86; director of nursing, LTC, 1988-99; nurse educator, 1990-99 at Delta College and currently, nurse manager of neuro-ortho-paedics at Covenant Medical Center.

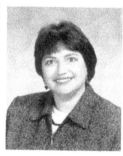

Earned her BS HCA at University of Michigan and MSN at Saginaw Valley State University. Professional activities are Sigma Theta Tau, MNA/ANA, NAON and AAUW.

Accomplishments include being listed in *Who's Who of America for Professional Managers;* published in *Michigan Nurse* (October 1966); a certified Board of Education member; past president, Bay Central Chapter; and poster presentation MNA Convention (October 1997).

Jane and her husband Rodney have two children, Trina and Shawn, and daughter-in-law, Connie.

MARGHERITA PROCACCINI CLARK, born in Toledo, OH, is a first generation Italian-American whose parents emigrated from Ancona, Italy in 1954 on the *Andrea Doria.* She became interested in healthcare during high school through service learning. She founded the Junior American Red Cross Council at Cardinal Stritch High School, active in the ARC Northwest, OH Chapter, and she was selected to represent all youth members at the ARC National Convention in Boston, MA in 1976. Coupled with volunteer work at the local hospital, this laid a foundation for a service career.

She began her college interests in the College of Pharmacy at the University of Toledo. After three years she made a career change to follow her heart to pursue a career in nursing. She completed her Diploma in Nursing in 1981 from Mercy School of Nursing, Toledo, OH and became licensed as a registered nurse. She received her BS in hospital management from the University of Toledo in 1987, became a certified critical care nurse (CCRN) in 1989, and completed her MSN at Michigan State University in 1999 with a specialty in geriatrics. She is a certified geriatric nurse practitioner.

Currently she is the Nursing Careers Department Chair at Lansing Community College where she has been instrumental in expanding the Career Ladder Nursing Program by 90% and offering fast track to RN programs for LPNs and paramedics, began a part-time RN Program, and developed and implemented Nurse Intern Programs for LPNs and RNs. In 2002, she successfully led the faculty team to achieve the highest level of accreditation award, eight years, through the National League for Nursing Accrediting Commission.

She holds multiple memberships in a variety of local, state, and national organizations, including the Michigan Nurses Association as a delegate and a Nominations Committee Representative. Additionally she is a parish nurse at St. Joseph Catholic Church in St. Johns. Recently she was nominated to the Michigan Board of Nursing.

She is married and lives with husband Dan in the country in St. Johns where they have resided since 1987.

RISA COLEMAN, born July 13, 1949 in Montgomery, AL. She holds both a master's of science degree in adult psychiatric nursing and a bachelor's of science in nursing, from Wayne State University. She is a current member of the Sigma Theta Tau Honor Society.

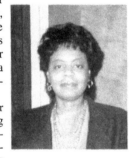

Her prior clinical nursing experiences include adult psychiatric nursing instructor; community health nursing and psychiatric staff nursing experience. She is currently the director of clinical services at a large outpatient Community Mental Health Agency serving over 75,000 persons with disabilities. Professional activities include membership in the Michigan Nursing Association and the American Psychiatric Nursing Association. She is also a member of Wayne State's Nursing Alumni.

She is married and has one daughter who recently graduated from the University of Michigan. Risa is dedicated to improving the delivery of health care to persons with mental illness and developmental disabilities.

DEBORAH BACH COLEY, born in Lansing, Michigan, received a BSN degree from the University of Michigan (UM) in 1987 and obtained her license to practice as

RN. She worked as a staff nurse on various units at UM, St Joseph Mercy, and Mott Children's Hospitals as well as in home health care in Ann Arbor.

In 1991 she received MPH and MSW degrees from UM. Her graduate internships included facilitating a support group for pregnant, drug addicted inmates, providing individual counseling to women in a residential substance abuse treatment program, and assisting in the design and grant writing for one of the nations first residential, substance abuse treatment programs for pregnant and postpartum women and their infants, as well as providing nursing care coordination for chronically ill children and public health analyst assistance for the BCBS of Western Pennsylvania Children's Caring Program.

She was the Michigan Senate Majority Policy Advisor from 1992-94 and Director of Government Affairs for the Michigan Nurses Association from 1994-96. She has three daughters and is actively involved in the health ministry at St. Francis of Assisi Catholic Church as well as the Michigan Nurses Association-Political Action Committee. She currently is a senior analyst at the Altarum Institute, where her work has included performing a literature review to identify nursing quality indicators for the American Nurses Association. She also chaired the Internet Prescribing Subcommittee of the 2000-01 Michigan Department of Consumer and Industry Affairs Task Force on Health Profession and the Internet.

ANN MARIE COLLINS, MA, MSN, RN, CS, was educated at The Jewish Hospital School of Nursing, Diploma; Wayne State University, BS in nursing; Wayne State University, MS in nursing/child and adolescent psychiatric and mental health; Wayne State University, MA in counseling education. She also holds ANCC Certification in child and adolescent psychiatric/mental health nursing and community/public health nursing.

Her research interests are health promotion and disease prevention for those with chronic mental illness and effects of family and community support in the prevention of alcohol abuse in adolescents.

Assignments include The Jewish Hospital of St. Louis, MO; Providence Hospital, South Field, MI; Holy Cross Hospital, Detroit, MI; Oakland County Health Division, Oakland County, MI; Wayne State University, Detroit, MI; clinical staff nurse, Field Public Health, supervisor, clinical instructor and assistant professor (clinical). Currently, she is teaching psychiatric and community health nursing at Wayne State University, Detroit, MI and is doctoral student in counseling edu-

cation also at Wayne State University. Her parents, Aloyes and Florence Wosmansky, were instrumental in influencing her to pursue a career in nursing.

KATHLEEN CONNORS, RN, born April 23, 1952, Milwaukee, WI. Earned her diploma in 1973 at Milwaukee County General Hospital School of Nursing.

Assignments include Med/Surg nursing, St. Mary's Hospital, Milwaukee, WI; ICU/CCLL St. Elizabeth's Hospital, Appleton, WI; small town hospital nursing, Baraga County Memorial Hospital, L'Anse; ICU, endoscopy, outpatient surgery and recovery room at Marquette General Hospital, Marquette, MI.

Awards: certified gastroenterology clinician, 1989-1994. She is listed in *Who's Who In American Nursing.* Kathleen is a member of Michigan Nurses Association, 1976 to present and a member of Society of Gastroenterology Nurses and Associates, 1988-91.

Kathleen and her husband Dale Timothy Connors have two children, Timothy and Jennifer.

MARK P. COOK, born Sept. 26, 1948, San Gabriel, CA. He earned his BSN at University of Vermont in 1980. Assignments include OR staff nurse, Medical Center Hospital of Vermont, 1980-83; assistant head nurse, OR Neurosurgery, 1983-85, Vermont; OR staff nurse, Borgess Medical Center, Kalamazoo, MI, 1985 to present.

Mark and his wife Mary (Chapman) have been married 33 years and have two sons, Peter and Jonathan.

JULIE COON, RN, MSN, EdD, earned her BSN from Grand Valley State Colleges in 1975, her MSN from Wayne State University in 1982 in women's health and her EdD from Western Michigan University in educational leadership in 1997. She was a faculty member at Ferris State University for 16 years before assuming her current position as

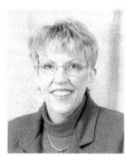

the academic department head for nursing and dental hygiene in 2001.

Dr. Coon has been active in MNA as a member of the Congress on Public Policy, the MNA PAC, as a delegate and is currently serving as chapter secretary of the Northern Great Lakes Chapter 2. She participated in the MNA task force to review the education rules of the Board of Nursing and recently served on the executive director search committee.

Dr. Coon was the 1994 recipient of the Carnegie Professor of the Year award, a

GVSU Distinguished Alumni in 1995 and was recently named as a finalist in the Nursing Excellence Awards for *Nurseweek* as an educator.

DOROTHY HELEN COYE, born June 9, 1916, Sturgis, MI. Earned diploma, Henry Ford Hospital School of nursing, Detroit, MI in 1938; BSN with distinction in 1963 and MSN in 1964, Wayne State University, College of Nursing.

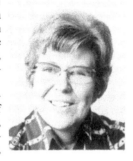

Assignments as staff nurse, head nurse, supervisor, assistant director, inservice education, Henry Ford Hospital, Detroit, MI, 1945-46, 1962; assistant director, associate director of nursing education, William Beaomont Hospital, Royal Oak, MI, 1967-83; U.S. Army Nurse Corps, 309th Gen. Hosp., Central Pacific Theater, U.S. Army of Occupation, Japan, 1945-46.

Member of American Nurses' Association, ANA Council on Continuing Education, Michigan Nurses Association, Sigma Theta Tau (Lambda Chapter), and Michigan Heart Association.

Dorothy has authored articles, editorials in nursing journals; contributed chapters in text book *The Process of Staff Development Components for Change;* and developed and tested tool for rating MNA continuing education programs. She was honored to be profiled in *Who's Who of American Women, Who's Who in Health Care* and *Who's Who in the Midwest* and was the subject of article in 1983 *Journal of Continuing Education in Nursing.* Dorothy received an invitation from World Health Organization to conduct a course in organizing continuing education in Bangladesh and has received Certificates of Appreciation from Oakland District Nurses Association, Michigan Nurses Association, Journal of Nursing Continuing Education Review Board, Oakland Community College Faculty.

Memorable experiences include world travels with Nomads, Inc.; being member of American Nurses Association tour of Peoples Republic of China in 1979; and participating in workshops throughout the USA to present revised standards in staff development.

Her family consists of parents, Charles and Harriet Coye; sister, Charlotte Coye; brother, Robert Coye; niece, Susan Coye Harris, LPN; nephew, Charles R. Coye and his wife Janis, RN PhD.

Dorothy is retired and enjoys her summer cottage at Klinger Lake, MI; traveling; and being active in community activities.

DONNA J. CRAIG, born Nov. 19, 1953, Detroit, MI. Earned her BSN in 1975 at University of Michigan School of Nursing (graduating cum laude) and JD in 1982 at Western New England College School of Law.

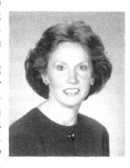

She started her nursing career as an aide at nursing homes and on a GYN floor at a local hospital while going to nursing school. After graduation she moved to Massachusetts and experienced "primary nursing" at Beth Israel Hospital. The most fulfilling aspect of nursing is the loving connection with patients in need.

Assignments at Beth Israel Hospital, Boston, MA, 1975-79, worked on a medical and cardiac care step-down unit, Springfield Hospital, Springfield, MA, 1979-82, worked on chronic care floor. At Beth Israel she started as staff nurse and was promoted to acting head nurse and while there, developed and designed EKG teaching manual for new graduate nurses.

From 2002 to present, Donna has served as secretary for the Southeast Chapter of the MNA. She also serves as nurse attorney in her own law firm and specializes in health care law, representing RNs and other health professionals and facilities and serves as arbitrator and mediator of health care and business disputes.

Donna married Barry Burrell in 1986 and they have one daughter Allison born in 1990.

MARGUERITE (ROBERTSON) CURTIS
see page 165

ANITA DACPANO DAUS, born in the Philippines and came to the U.S. via the Exchange Visitors Program. She is married to a professional engineer and they are blessed with three children who are all professionals.

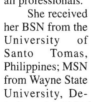

She received her BSN from the University of Santo Tomas, Philippines; MSN from Wayne State University, Detroit; and a PhD from Michigan State University, MI.

She was a nursing instructor, then assistant director at Hurley Medical Center, Flint, MI. She is a professor at Mott Community College, Flint, MI, and she served as Dean of the School of Health and Human Sciences after being chairperson of the division of nursing.

She is a member of the Board of Directors of the MNA representing the Bay

Central Chapter. She served as vice chairperson of the Michigan Board of Nursing and was NLNAC program evaluator of associate degree programs in nursing. She was Flint District Nurse of the Year.

SALLY DECKER, born in Mitchell, SD and professor of nursing and former captain in Army. Earned her BSN, University of Maryland, Baltimore; MSN, University of North Carolina, Chapel Hill; and PhD, University of Michigan, Ann Arbor.

Awards include Robert Woods Johnston Scholarship, Phi Kappa Phi, Sigma Theta Tau, and awards for teaching and scholarship at SVSU. Sally is a former member of MNA Congress on Nursing Practice, Cabinet on Nursing Research.

Currently she is faculty member at Saginaw Valley State University.

AMY (BRESLIN) DELANEY was born in Lansing, MI. She started her nursing career in 11th grade, working co-op after school as a certified nurses aide. She continued nursing classes and was inspired by one of her instructors, Violet Seymour. Through relentless efforts, she received her LPN in 1992 from Grand Rapids Junior

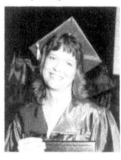

College and started working in the orthoneuro unit at Sparrow Hospital in Lansing, MI. Continuing on in her career, she graduated magna cum laude from Lansing Community College in 1997 with her best friend, Shannon French. Together, they continued on at Grand Valley State University, and in 2003 obtained a BSN degree.

She is married, has two children and is a member of Holy Family in Ovid, MI. Today, she works at Sparrow Regional Children's Center and will start part-time as a pediatric clinical instructor for LCC. In 2004, she plans to pursue her PNP degree at GVSU.

MARIA A. DELINE, RN, born Aug. 26, 1976, Lansing, MI. Earned her associates degree in applied sciences from Lansing Community College. She graduated Phi Theta Kappa, Summa Cum Laude.

Marci is currently taking pre-requisite classes for University of Michigan's master's program. Her assignments include Orthopedic/Neurology Unit at Sparrow Hospital in Lansing, MI; part-time and family practice – per diem. Also active in pain management liaison for hospital unit.

She and her husband Carl have one daughter, Natasha.

JULIE ANN (HAMILTON) DEROSSETT, born in Washington, DC and became interested in nursing when she was only 15 years old. She decided to become an RN following after her great-grandmother who was a small town (Robbinsville, NC) midwife. She delivered babies or provided other medical treatment for a sack of flour or a couple of chickens.

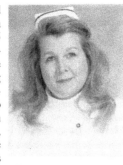

Julie graduated with honors with an applied art and science degree in 2000 and obtained her license to practice as an RN. She is employed by the University of Michigan. She is a dedicated nurse on a surgical transplant, GI and urology floor. She has received many supers for her caring work toward her patients.

She is a Christian who believes in the many miracles of prayer. She has one daughter, Julie Marie; her mother and father, Robert and Dawn Hamilton; one sister, Dawn Hamilton Goll and four nieces and nephews: Ashley, Alex, Victoria and Sierra. Her greatest passion in life is for animals.

She has three dogs: Dopey, Lucky and Max.

BETTY DICE, born Dec. 19, 1955, Lansing, MI. She was a RN and staff nurse at Lapeer Regional Hospital and is currently a charge nurse of a 20 bed telemetry unit at LRH.

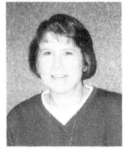

Earned her LPN from Northwestern Community College in 1975 and RN from Mott Community College in 1988.

She received E&GW Award on two separate occasions and assisted the nurses at LRH to become organized under MNA.

Betty is married with two grown daughters.

LAVONNE R. DIGBY, RN, born April 12, 1954 in Jackson, MI. She has associates degree in applied arts and science, Jackson Community College, 1976; bachelor's degree in management and organizational development in 2000, Spring Arbor College.

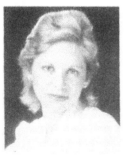

She has worked as hospital staff nurse, 1976-91, med/surg., coronary care, operating room, newborn nursery, post partum; 1991-2004, Home Health Care and physicians office. She has worked as an RN mostly in the Lansing area.

Compassion for other people's pain inspired her to be a nurse. Her hero was her aunt who was an RN and joined the military in WWII. The women in her family felt a duty in helping others and being good Christians. Proverbs 31 also inspired Lavonne.

The hours are long and there are many exhausting tasks to be performed in the health care profession, but it is a most rewarding experience getting to know the patients and helping to make them feel better. The patients come from all walks of life and with a wide variety of health care concerns. She has learned much from them.

Lavonne and Robert Digby, MD, married in 1983. Their son, Philip, was born in 1985. Lavonne is currently working for Michigan Plastic Surgery, staff nurse as a circulator in outpatient surgery and makes many home care visits, post-op, for the physician.

Received Certificate of Participation, 1989-99. Enrolled in the Nurses Health Study I & II to further the knowledge of women's health issues on behalf of the Harvard School of Public Health and the Channing Laboratory at Brigham and Women's Hospital.

CINDY BOROVOY DISKIN, RN, MSN, APRN, BC, Adult Nurse Practitioner, Board Certified, the West Bloomfield resident is determined to offer an alternative to traditional medical care, care that has become increasingly more rushed and impersonal. As the number of options for treatment of many conditions has increased, many

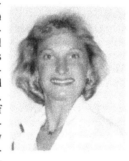

people are finding that they want more time to discuss the best way to manage, or prevent, health problems. Cindy wants to give her patients more time.

As a board certified nurse practitioner, she is breaking new ground by hanging out her own shingle in Southfield, and she specializes in providing counseling and education about health maintenance and disease prevention. She can work with a patient's doctor, taking time to provide patients with the information they need to manage a specific condition such as asthma, migraine headaches, osteoporosis, hypertension, and high cholesterol, to name a few. Alternatively, she can provide "one-stop shopping," including comprehensive medical management of acute and chronic problems, along with health counseling and skills training. At Ms. Diskin's new practice,

called Adult Primary Care Associates, all of the services found in most doctors' offices are available, including x-rays and lab work.

People will often start with, "This is a stupid question, but…" and then go on to ask something really important, such as "How can I lower my cholesterol? Or "My mother had breast cancer, I'm concerned that I am at risk, what do I look out for?" Says Diskin, "Good health care means providing time to answer all questions, and of course, there are no stupid questions." Most importantly, the key to being a good nurse practitioner is being a good listener!

People ask, what is a nurse practitioner? A nurse practitioner is a registered nurse who has advanced training and clinical experience. Nurse practitioners take classes in pharmacology, pathophysiology and health assessment. Before going into practice, nurse practitioners must log a minimum of 500 supervised hours working with patients, complete a master's degree and pass an exam in their specialty administered by the American Academy of Nurse Practitioners.

The role was first developed in the 1980s to serve underserved populations, but nurse practitioners now work in a variety of specialties and in general practice. They can be found in private practice, group practices and in hospitals. In Michigan, NPs may work independently, but most have a collaborative agreement with a physician which allows them to write prescriptions. Ms. Diskin is the second nurse practitioner owned business in the state of Michigan. Ms. Diskin has agreements with Drs. Larry Dell and Barbara Cingel. Dr. Dell is affiliated with Huron Valley-Sinai Hospital in Commerce and Dr. Cingel is a hospitalist at William Beaumont Hospital in Royal Oak.

Besides offering health care with an emphasis on "care," Ms. Diskin is especially excited to be able to offer visits to patient's homes, or to extended care residences, for those people who are not able to drive. This service should be greatly appreciated by grown children who struggle to get their home-bound parents to doctor's office appointments. Laboratory services will be available on home visits, as Ms. Diskin is a proficient phlebotomist after years working in intensive care. She brings to her practice her many years of hospital training in medical/critical care and her last seven years working in a private practice in internal medicine. She not only takes great pride in caring for her patients and their families, she endlessly finds time for her very supportive, caring husband, Jeffrey and their beautiful family of four children: Joshua (age 17 years), Michael and Rachel (15-year-old twins) and Jacob (12 years old).

She received her BSN at Wayne State University School of Nursing in Detroit in 1984, worked at Sinai Hospital for years, then went into a private practice for almost seven years with premier internists as an advanced practice nurse. She obtained both her MSN in adult chronic illness at Madonna University in Livonia, MI and her Certification as an Adult Nurse Practitioner a couple of years later. She is actively involved in many nursing organizations, such as Sigma Theta Tau, and Michigan Council of Nurse Practitioners (MICNP), as well as offering free educational seminars, being actively involved with medical/nursing research and mentoring student nurse practitioners.

LYNDA DOLPHUS, MSN, RN, Instructor, born July 14, 1959, Detroit, MI. Earned her LPN diploma in 1986, JTPA Practical Nurse School; associate in applied sciences in 1993, Wayne County Community College; BSN in 1999 and MSN in 2001, University of Phoenix; and in 2003, RA in the Trainer Certification, state of Michigan.

Background includes supervision, diabetic nurse educator, ambulatory care, managed care, med/surg, geratrics and critical care.

She received Outstanding Employee Recognition Certificate (The Wellness Plan), Exceptional Care Giver Certificate (St. John's Hospital), and in 2002 was selected to attend Diabetic Educator Forum in San Diego, CA.

A former member of Henry Ford Health System JCAHO Team and Safety Committee and has been a member of MNA for three years.

Married with two sons, age 24 and 15, she is currently part-time instructor and homemaker.

ROBBI DUDA, MS, RN, BC, was born Roberta Ann Paas in Grand Haven, MI in 1956. She decided to become a nurse because she felt nursing made one a wonderful mother.

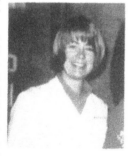

While working as an LPN (Muskegon Community College in 1979), she went back to school and subsequently worked many night and weekend shifts to get her additional degrees. As a BSN student she eventually became the president of University of Michigan's Nursing Student Organization and was inducted into the Rho Chapter of Sigma Theta Tau International Nursing Honor Society in 1985.

She joined the MNA and ANA immediately upon graduation and volunteered in many positions in the organization to include the state level Board of Directors, Finance Committee, Political Action Committee, and on the local level as delegate and the union treasurer. Presently she is an AANC Board Certified Gerontological Nurse and has also worked for many years in psychiatry at the Michigan Department of Mental Health and at the University of Michigan.

After completing her MS in community health (U of M, 1997), she started her own independent business called Nurses Foot Care & Massage Services. Her service objectives, in addition to providing excellent foot care, included individualized risk assessment, health, safety, and grief counseling and teaching people how to be wise and assertive health care consumers. Her website is at www.NursesCare.net.

In 2000 she became the president Michigan Nurses in Business Association and started a second business, NFCS Associates Services, LLC. This business provides an innovative online business training program for RNs, a newsletter, and an on-going support to independent RN business owners through a corporate intranet on the internet.

She currently is in the process of writing, *Foot Notes from the Foot Care Nurse,* and loves family, friends and cats, plus yoga, ballroom dancing, bungy jumping and golf. Her future goal is to build, manage and live in a small, elegant assisted living retirement home in Ann Arbor, MI.

PEGGY ANNE DUTCHER, RN, ADN, BSN, born Sept. 19, 1941, Bad Axe, MI. Earned her ADN in May 1975, College of the Ablemarle and BSN in 1988, Saginaw Valley State College.

Assignments as charge nurse 11-7 shift, North Carolina, 1975-77; charge nurse 11-7 shift, 1977-82; 3-11 charge nurse until

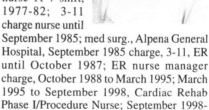

September 1985; med surg., Alpena General Hospital, September 1985 charge, 3-11, ER until October 1987; ER nurse manager charge, October 1988 to March 1995; March 1995 to September 1998, Cardiac Rehab Phase I/Procedure Nurse; September 1998-January 2004.

Received Literary Award for library personnel in May 1977; was Employee of Month in 1988 and in 1993; received Letter of Appreciation from PT in 1993.

Peggy is ANA member, ENA member, MNA member, staff council treasurer Unit One, president Unit II, CHF teaching program, Ethics Committee member and Red Cross volunteer.

Her husband passed away in November 1995. She has four children: Allen, Cheryl, Douglas and Lynnette. Three of her children attended college and youngest son made chief after 21 years in Navy. Her youngest daughter is a nurse.

She is currently trying to expand her rug weaving business, catching up on reading and helping oldest grandson with college. She is still on Ethics Committee.

FAYE A. (SIERSMA) EBACH, BSN, MSN, RN, Nursing Faculty, Division Chair, born April 8, 1932, Detroit, MI. Earned her BSN, University of Michigan in 1955; MSN, Wayne State University in 1977; graduate of National Community College Leadership Program for Deans and Chairs (NCC Chair Academy), 1992-93.

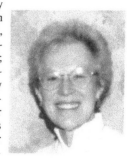

Assignments include University of Michigan, Ann Arbor, staff nurse; William Beaumont Hospital, Royal Oak/Staff Nurse; Midland Hospital, Midland/Staff Nurse; Delta College, University Center/Nursing Faculty, Chair Nursing Division.

Received the Sigma Theta Tau, Theta Chi Chapter Excellence in Nursing Award. Other activities include member Sigma Theta Tau; former treasurer Theta Chi Chapter; member, National League for Nursing; Michigan League for nursing; former MLN board member; MNA/Bylaws Committee member; former Finance and Nominations Committee member; former member Michigan Community College Nursing Directors Association.

Married 50 years, they are both retired. They reared a family of four children, all of whom have graduated from college, have successful careers and rearing their own families. Most memorable experience was having an impact on student's educational development.

Faye is still active in MNA and serves on Bylaws Committee; she is active in genealogy research, produces and edits newsletter for Midland Genealogical Society, travels a great deal throughout the USA and world, spends time with her children and eight grandchildren. She travels annually with children and grandchildren (two families live and work in various parts of U.S.)

WANDA ELOISE (ROBINSON) EDWARDS, born in Little Rock, AR. Her mother, Rosetta Robinson, is credited with lovingly and skillfully guiding her toward a career in nursing. Her mother was an educator. She stressed the importance of a college education and repeatedly recommended nursing as a career option.

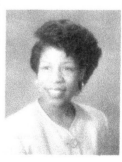

Wanda received a BSN in 1973 and an MSN in 1990 from Wayne State University. Her professional memberships include ANA, Chi Eta Phi

Sorority Inc., The American Psychiatric Nurses Association and Sigma Theta Tau.

She is a psychiatric mental health nurse practitioner and founder, CEO of Health and Business Consultants. She provides counseling, consultation and evidence based staff development programs promoting healthy lifestyles, and healthy prosperous business practices.

God and family are most important. Her husband, Willie, daughter Sherri Collins, son-in-law Terrance Collins and grandson Cameron Wade Collins along with other family and friends, add immeasurable joy to her life.

CAROLYN EPPLETT, RN, MSN, CS, FNP, earned her BSN in 1973, University of Michigan; MSN in 1986, major in advanced medical/surgical nursing, minors in nursing administration and education, Wayne State University; Post Master's Certificate Program, Family Nurse Practitioner, 1998, Michigan State University.

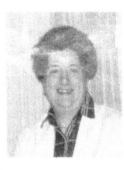

A family nurse practitioner at Health Delivery, Inc., Community Health Center, she enjoyed over 30 years of active nursing, working in critical care, home care, QI, management, education, preceptor for SVSU FNP program and mentor for aspiring nurses.

Awards include Saginawian of the Year, January 2002 and Outstanding Nurse of the Year, Bay Central Chapter, MNA in May 1997.

Professional Accomplishments: 1999-present, Certification Family Nurse Practitioner, ANA; 1992-97, Certification Nursing Administration, Advanced, ANA; 1980-96, CCRN, American Association of Critical Care Nurses.

Professional Activities: MNA, Member of Congress on Nursing & Health Care Economics, Treasurer, East Central District; Founding Member, Saginaw Valley College Honor Society in Nursing; Sigma Theta Tau, member since 1972, Theta Chi Chapter member vice-president, Theta Chi; member of Mid-Michigan Nurse Practitioner Network and Michigan Council of Nurse Practitioners.

Carolyn dedicates her career and successes to her life partner, Paul Epplett, who died unexpectedly in February 2003 and who blessed her with three children: Christopher, Courtney and Nicole

NAOMI E. ERVIN, PhD, RN, APRN, BC, FAAN, born in Lincoln Park, MI, realized her interest in nursing at the young age of 5 years. She holds degrees in nursing, public health nursing and education from the University of

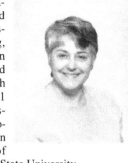

Michigan. Her career has included practice, administration, teaching, and research in public health and community health nursing. In 2001 she became assistant dean and associate professor in the College of Nursing, Wayne State University.

She is a member of Sigma Theta Tau International, the American Academy of Nursing, and Delta Omega (public health honor society). She served on the MNA Board of Directors, MNA committees, and several district positions. In Illinois she was president of the Chicago Nurses Association and a member of the INA Board of Directors. In 2000-04 she served on the ANA Congress on Nursing Practice and Economics and on the ANCC Commission on Certification.

CHERYL ARTZ FEENSTRA, born and reared in Holland, MI, decided to become a nurse while in the sixth grade. In 1972 she graduated magna cum laude from the University of Michigan also joining Sigma Theta Tau International. Beginning years were spent in public health and orthopedic nursing. A 1979 MSN degree from Wayne State University in obstetric nursing led to teaching part time for 10 years at Grand Valley State University. While there she was instrumental in initiating a chapter of Sigma Theta Tau and became its first president. In 1989 she joined the nursing faculty at Calvin College, rising from assistant to full professor and most recently serving as chairperson of the department. A PhD in family ecology was awarded by Michigan State University in 1996. She has been an active member of MNA since college graduation, serving on many committees, chapter offices and as a delegate to many MNA conventions.

LORENE R. FISCHER served as Dean of the College of Nursing at Wayne State University from 1977-89. Prior to becoming Dean, she was a professor and Director of WSU's Undergraduate Program in Nursing. She chaired the Department of Psychiatric Nursing from 1957-75.

A Fellow in the American Academy of Nursing since 1977, she is also a member of Sigma Theta Tau. She served in leadership capacities for professional organizations including the Michigan Association of Colleges of

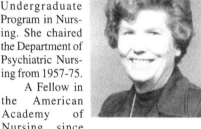

Nursing, the American Academy of Nursing, the Michigan Nurses Association and the American Nurses Association.

She served on the board of directors of Blue Cross Blue Shield of Michigan from 1990-2003. Service on other boards of directors includes the Greater Detroit Council for the Blind and the Visiting Nurses Association of Metropolitan Detroit.

She consulted throughout the United States and globally for the World Health Organization and other organizations in Africa, Europe, Australia and the Middle-East. A recognized leader in the areas of psychiatric-mental health nursing and nursing education, she published numerous articles on emotionally disturbed children and the development of the nursing profession and marketing of nursing education.

Dean Fischer currently resides in Dearborn with her husband Heinz. Her daughter, Susan Warner, lives in Arlington, VA.

DIANE FLATLEY, RN, BSN, born Oct. 14, 1954 in Detroit, MI. Earned her BSN at Michigan State University in 1976. Assignments include Sparrow Hospital, Lansing PACU, 1989-2004; Acute Pain Service, 1997-2000, Crittenton Hospital Orthopedics, 1978-79; ICU 1980-86, Bon Secours, Grosse Pointe, MI, 1976-78.

Memorable experience was working under the direction of the anesthesiology group and helping manage epidurals and achieve effective pain control as a member of Acute Pain Service.

Diane received Honorable Mention Nurse of Year, Sparrow Hospital in 2002. Member of CCRN, 1983-89; ACLS, 1984 to present; and PALS, 2002 to present.

Diane married John in 1976 and they have three children: Ellen, Erin and Eric. She is currently working in a busy PACU, caring for all ages.

MARGARET M. FLATT, born in Detroit, MI to parents who valued education and responsible citizenship through community service. Participating in family care of her grandmother, she learned of the challenges and satisfactions accompanying the caring role.

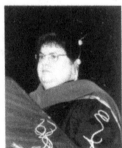

Margaret obtained a BSN from Mercy College of Detroit, a MA in nursing from the University of Iowa, and a PhD from Michigan State University. While in the Army Nurse Corps, she served in the Vietnam War. Margaret worked in hospitals, public health, and academia.

Leadership positions include chairperson of the Midland County Board of Health, and member of the Board of Directors of MNA and the Committee on Bylaws of ANA. Honors include induction into Sigma Theta Tau, and recognition for service by the Michigan Nurses Association, her local MNA and Sigma Theta Tau chapters, and the Faculty Association of Saginaw Valley State University.

SUSAN L. FOGARTY, born in Ludington, MI and grew up in Muskegon. She received a BSN from Mercy College of Detroit, MSN from Wayne State University in Community Health Nursing and Primary Health Care Certification from Case-Western Reserve University.

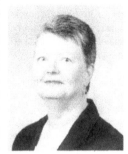

Professional memberships include Sigma Theta Tau, the American Public Health Association and the Michigan Nurses Association In MNA she most recently served on the Congress for Nursing and Health Care Economics and President of Chapter 3. In 2003 she received the Bertha Lee Culp Human Rights Award for advocacy for the glbt community.

Susan is an associate professor of nursing at Ferris State University. Previously she was employed as an FNP and in public health in Detroit and Texas.

Susan's mother, who was a nurse's aide, inspired her career with her talk of her own unfulfilled desire to be a nurse and her respect for her nurse co-workers.

DIANE PORRETTA FOX, born in Detroit, MI, became interested in healthcare while caring for her mother at home with a malignant brain tumor. Science and teaching have also been an active interest. She was a member of the initial second career program at the University of Michigan School of Nursing. In 1997 this class graduated 13

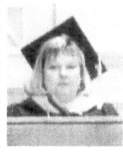

BSN students who had previously obtained BS or BA degrees. Nola Pender, RN, PhD, started the class together at a Sunday brunch held in her home in February 1996. Jan Lee, RN, PhD, led this group through to graduation.

Diane is a member of the American Association of Critical Care Nurses, Transcultural Nursing Society, American Association of Respiratory Care and the University of Michigan Nursing Alumni

Society. She became a member of the Rho chapter of Sigma Theta Tau International Honor Society while attending the University of Michigan School of Nursing. Currently she is vice president of the Eta Rho Chapter while attending Eastern Michigan University School of Nursing Master's Degree in Nursing Science program.

Awards include the following peer awards from U of M School of Nursing, "perseverance" and "clinical performance." She was selected as the MSN 2003 Outstanding Graduate student at Eastern Michigan University. She was awarded the Sigma Theta Tau - Eta Rho member research award for 2003.

She obtained an AS, Honors in Respiratory Therapy in 1978 from Washtenaw Community College. Then a BA Magna Cum Laude in general studies with a business concentration from Siena Heights College in 1989. A BSN Magna Cum Laude in Nursing from the University of Michigan in 1997. Teaching in Health Care Systems certificate from Eastern Michigan University in 2001. She plans to complete the research study thesis and graduate with an MSN in December 2003 from Eastern Michigan University.

Diane plans to continue her education toward a doctorate. She maintains her love of science and teaching. She is an adjunct faculty lecturer for Monroe County Community College and Washtenaw Community College, teaching nursing students. She is a per diem staff registered nurse for the University of Michigan Extracorporeal Membrane Oxygenation department. She also teaches respiratory therapy students and is an asthma educator. She has served as a Cardiopulmonary Director where she developed and initiated smoking cessation programs, pulmonary rehabilitation, and occupational health lung screening.

She has two adult children who make her proud and a loving husband of 28 years. She is a Master Gardener volunteer, Big Sister volunteer, and board member of the Lenawee County March of Dimes.

SUZETTE DEE FRANKLIN, born Oct. 21, 1958, Escanaba, MI. She has worked in Home Health for nine years, intensive care for four years, coronary care for six years, intermediate care for two years, all as staff RN at Marquette General Hospital, Marquette, MI.

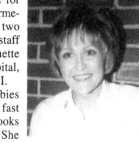

Her hobbies are exercise, fast cars, good books and movies. She enjoys life and meeting new people daily. The ability to help others through nursing is an experience that no other job can ever match.

She earned her degree through Northern Michigan University and graduated with bachelor's of nursing. Suzette currently works for Marquette General Hospital in the CCU/ICU.

Suzette has three beautiful children: Jessie Dee Miller, Sandie Lee Miller and James Daniel Miller.

KAREN A. FRATTO, born Sept. 27, 1952, Wayne County. She graduated from Madonna University with a BSN degree when she was 50 years old. She is very proud to have made it considering all the hassles and obstacles she encountered along the way to her goal.

Assigned to ICU, Neuro at University of Michigan, she enjoys being an ICU and ER nurse and teaching CPR.

Karen is the mother of four sons: Michael, Robert, Brian and Richard, and the grandmother of four.

ALTA SOMSEL ZAHN FREARS, born March 4, 1939, to an eight member logging family in Brethren, MI. As a youngster she wanted to be a nurse which her parents nurtured. She graduated from Norman-Dickson High School in Brethren and attended Muskegon's Hackley Hospital School of Nursing where she graduated as a di-

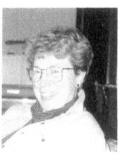

ploma nurse in 1960. She complimented her education by graduating in 1977 from John Wesley College, in Owosso, with a BA in behavioral science. In 1982 she became ANA certified as a psychiatric/mental health nurse, which she continued until her 1998 retirement. In 1985 she received her Social Worker license.

She joined MNA as a student and is a life member. She was active in the former Shiawassee District. She served on MNA's Continuing Education Committee and facilitated the merger of Shiawassee District with Genessee.

Her career experiences include medical/surgical, psychiatric in-patient, volunteer instructor of Red Cross Home Nursing, manager of a blood bank, taught a health class for the public school and private duty nursing. She established the Shiawassee Alliance for the mentally ill and continues an AMI membership. While working at Shiawassee Community Mental Health, Atrium/Kalkaska CMH and Grand Traverse CMH, she served as a client services manager, assertive community treatment team leader, group home trainer, OBRA nursing assessor and the coordinator of Medication Clinic. She retired from GT CMH in 1998. She has been an active member of the Harvard Medical School Nurses' Health Study since 1976. In 1978 she went on a mission trip to Haiti where she worked with Haitian nurses in outpatient clinics.

She and husband, Rob, live in Traverse City. She has two daughters, two stepsons (who are all married) and eight grandchildren. She serves on the Senior Advisory Council at Northwestern Michigan College, sings in her church choir, enjoys reading, traveling, writing, sewing, gardening, biking, cross-country skiing, volunteering at her daughter's stores and people.

LINDA K. FROST, Charge Nurse, born June 18, 1954. Received her education at Ann Arbor Practical Nurse Education Center and Jackson Community College Transition Program.

A charge nurse at Bixby Medical Center, she has received the Ambassabor Award and is active in various care committees.

Linda and her husband Jack have two daughters, six sons, 10 grandchildren, two horses, three dogs and three cats.

LOIS W. GAGE, born March 8, 1922, Ipswich, MA. Earned her BS at Simmons College in 1949; MA at Teachers College, Columbia University, 1957; PhD, U of M in 1972; certificate/reg. St. Elizabeth's School of Nursing, Brighton, MA in 1943.

Assignments include 1973-91, professor of nursing, U of M; 1963-91, assoc. prof. of nursing, WSU; 1963-69, asst. prof. of nursing, NYU; 1958-61, MH Cons. VNSNY; 1957-58, supervisor, Pittsburgh Health Dept.; 1949-52, staff nurse, New Haven, CN; 1944-46, U.S. Navy Nurse Reserve, LTJG.

In 1996 she received the Academic Women's Caucus Power Award; Sigma Thete Tau Excellence in Nursing Award, 1989; MH Section Award, APNA, 1983; and Fellow AAN, 1977.

Other activities include leadership roles in Mental Health Section, APHA (1977-87) initiator of Psychiatric/Mental Health Conference Group, MNA, 1963-65; Consultant to PAHO and WHO and various schools of nursing in Europe, Latin America and Asia; initiated community clinical experiences for graduate students at NYU in psychiatric mental health nursing at NYU, prior to the passage of the Community Mental Health Legislation and developed the role and the curriculum to prepare primary care/nurse practitioner graduate students; was the first chair of the International Committee at the School of Nursing, U of M and participated with the University of Michigan Advisory Committee for the Institute of International Affairs.

Lois is the mother of two children, Nancy Gage-Lindner and John. Currently, she is retired and writing her memoirs.

NANCY M. GAGNON, born Oct. 18, 1942, Hazel Park, MI. Graduated in May 1963 from Detroit Practical Nurse Program and licensed as an LPN in November 1963. She worked at William Beaumont Hospital, Royal Oak, MI, 1963-66; St. Mary's Hospital, Livonia, MI, 1966-72; Cheboygan Memorial Hospital (CHM), Cheboygan, MI, 1972 to present.

Nancy returned to school in 1987 and graduated from North Central Community College in 1989 with an ADN and began working as an RN in November 1989 at CMH. She returned to school through Lake Superior State University in Sault Saint Marie, MI and graduated with BSN in December 1997 and continued working at CMH. Since July 2002 she has worked as manager of emergency services and urgent care at CMH.

Married 40 years, she had three children and three grandchildren. Active in MNA since 1989 on staff council, past president of District and officer in Chapter 2. She is currently serving as chair of Congress on Nurse Practice Congress representing Chapter 2. Also active in her church, local community activities and sings with several community groups.

RITA MUNLEY GALLAGHER, PHD, RN, serves as Senior Policy Fellow at the American Nurses Association (ANA) in Washington, DC. As such, she is charged with identifying, researching, analyzing, conducting, writing, coordinating and reporting on health policy activities related to ANA priorities. In this 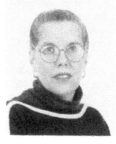 role, she prepares and provides input for development of policy statements and legislative testimony for the association.

Prior to coming to ANA, Dr. Gallagher had over 10 years experience in education, first at Oakland University in Rochester, as a tenured associate professor in the School of Nursing and lastly at Dominican College of San Raphel, CA where she directed the School of Nursing. Both her MSN in community health nursing and her PhD, in applied sociology, are from Wayne State University in Detroit.

In addition to the Michigan Nurses Association, Gallagher is a member of numerous professional organizations including APHA, where she has been elected to the Governing Council representing public health nursing. She currently serves on the Board of Directors of the American Medical Directors Association Foundation.

Dr. Gallagher is a Virginia Henderson Fellow of Sigma Theta Tau International. She has published in numerous peer-reviewed journals and presented world-wide on a variety of topics including care of the elderly and others in need of long term care, HIV/AIDS, client satisfaction with health care and health care reform.

MARIE F. GUTOWSKI GATES, PHD, MSN, BSN, RN, Marie holds two major institutions as primary in shaping her professional nursing career: Wayne State University (WSU) and Visiting Nurse Association (VNA) of Metropolitan Detroit. Her three degrees were obtained from WSU. Following the receipt of her BSN, Marie's first nursing position was as public health nurse at VNA where she subsequently served as field teacher, supervisor, district director, and education director.

She served as a faculty member in the Department of Public Health Nursing at WSU after obtaining her master's degree. After receiving her PhD in 1988, Marie held faculty positions at Eastern Michigan University, University of Tennessee-Memphis, and University of Missouri-Kansas City. Since 2000 she has been professor and director of the Western Michigan University Bronson School of Nursing.

Throughout her career, Marie has characterized herself a public health nurse and a teacher with special interests in transcultural nursing and care of persons who are dying and their families. She has published manuscripts and books in such areas as care and cure in hospital and hospice settings, needs of young caregivers of persons with cancer and other chronic diseases, theory in public health nursing, and qualitative research.

Marie's professional career as a nurse has been strongly supported by her husband of 40 years, George Gates; daughter Susan Gates (husband Jonathan Rho); and son Michael Gates (wife Amy Randel) and grandchildren, Madeleine and Nathaniel Gates.

BEVERLY GAUDETTO, RN, Staff Nurse, born July 28, 1960, Escanaba, MI. Earned her BSN at NMU, Marquette, MI, and work has worked at Dickinson County Memorial Hospital, 1983 to present. Worked at Marquette Home Health, 1989-90.

Activities include discharge planning, cardiac rehab, diabetic education, pediat- 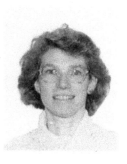 rics, medical floor staff nurse and weekend charge nurse. Currently ACU staff nurse.

Beverly and John have been married 23 years and have four children: Phillip, Angela, Matthew and Jacob.

MARIANNE GEORGE, RN, BSN, Clinical Nurse Educator, Pediatrics/PICU, born March 28, 1960, Dearborn, MI and earned her BSN at Michigan State University. Worked at Sparrow Hospital, Lansing, MI since 1982. She was assistant department manager, PICU, for 12 years.

Activities include Training Center coordinator, Sparrow Health System, Certified Pediatric Nurse (CPN), CCRN (prior), PALS instructor, regional faculty, instructor trainer.

Marianne and Greg have been married 18 years and have three daughters: Ariel, Lilly and Grace. She currently works part time for Sparrow in nursing education and is a training center coordinator for Sparrow Health System.

CYNTHIA J. GERSTENLAUER,

Adult/Gerontological Nurse Practitioner, MSN, APRN, BC, born Dec. 25, 1953, Northville, MI.
She earned her BSN at Madonna University, Livonia, MI; MSN at Wayne State University, Detroit, MI; and Specialist Certificate Aging, Institute of Geronology. Worked at Troy Internal Medicine, Troy, MI.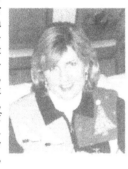

Activities include instructor, educational specialist, geriatric education, Center of Michigan; chair, Practice Committee of NCGNP; president, Great Lakes Chapter, NCGNP. She received Outstanding Gerontological Nurse of the Year, MNA, in 1991.

Currently, teaching and counseling for diabetes management, lipids, weight management, osteoporosis and geriatrics.

Cynthia and her husband Michael have two sons, Nicholas and Alexander.

MARY ANN GERWOLDS, RN, born

Oct. 1, 1954, Flint, MI. Earned her associate degree of nursing at Mott Community College. She has worked 27 years at Lapeer Regional Hospital and has RN experience in various areas.
Awarded Employee of the Month, she is active with RN Staffing Committee and is a member of MNA.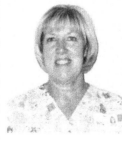

Mary Ann is still working at LRH, presently in OR recovery room.

Married 28 years, she has two sons, one brother, one sister and parents, all living in Davison.

LORA ANN GIBBS, Clinical Nurse I, born March 2, 1969, Kincheloe AFB, Kinross, MI. Earned BS in sports medicine, Eastern Michigan University in 1990; BSN at Eastern Michigan University in 2001.

Married, she is currently attending University of Michigan-Flint, working towards a master's degree in anesthesia.

Activities include Sigma Theta Tau Honor Society of Nursing, 1999-present and student member American Association of Nurse Anesthetists.

CYNTHIA ARCHER-GIFT, Chief Nurse Consultant, born Port-of-Spain, Trinidad. She is a graduate of Wayne State University with a PhD in higher education and a minor in psychiatric nursing administration, Education Specialist Certificate in Educational Administration and Supervision. She has a master's and 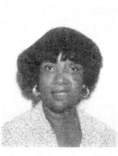 bachelors in nursing from University of Detroit-Mercy, RN, and Certificate in Midwifery.

Cynthia has held the following positions: Nurse-midwife in Scotland prior to immigrating to the U.S.; supervisor, Lafayette Clinic; director of nursing for Dept. of Mental Health Psychiatric Emergency Services program; psychiatric nurse surveyor centers for Medicare/Medicaid Services; nurse consultant, Division of Licensing and Monitoring; chief nurse consultant, Central Office, MDCH; consultant to Chief Nursing Officer Ministry of Republic of Trinidad and Tobago.

She received outstanding Faculty of the Year Award, 2001 from University of Phoenix; Outstanding Psychiatric Nurse of the Year MNA, 1989; nominee, Florence Nightingale annual Excellence in Nursing Award, 1995, 2000; Sigma Theta Tau International Award, 1999; Shelton Tappes Community Services Award from Detroit Area Agency on Aging; Appreciation Award, Detroit Black Nurses Association, 1990; International Nursing Award, Ministry of Health Government of Trinidad and Tobago, 1994; Commendation, Michigan Dept. of Mental Health, 1989); Elizabeth Carnegie Award for Doctoral Studies, 1990; Appreciation Award Women of Wayne Alumni, 1990; Minority Scholarship Center for Ethics and Humanities in the life sciences, 1994.

Other activities include Michigan representative to American Nurses Association House of Delegates, 2003; appointed to Curriculum Revision Committee, University of Phoenix-MI Campus, 1999; member of MNA; American Nurses Association; American Psychiatric Nurses Association; Caribbean Nurses Organization; American

Association of Nurse Practitioners; National League of Nursing; Sigma Theta Tau International Honor Society (Lambda Chapter); University of Detroit-Mercy.

She was appointed to Lead Faculty Graduate Nursing Students University of Phoenix, Michigan Campus (2004); appointed to Board of Directors, Detroit Central Cities Community Mental Health for 1982-86; board of directors, Detroit Agency on Aging, 1992-97; reviewer American Journal of Psychiatric Nursing, and she has a number of articles published in nursing journals.

Cynthia is a volunteer to Manna Soup Kitchen, St. Vincent De Paul Free Health Clinic and Adopt Senior Citizen. She is married to Fernandes and they have one son, Anthony.

She continues to work tirelessly with nursing students serving as a mentor. She enjoys conducting national surveys for Centers for Medicare/Medicaid Services and providing community services as needed to her parish community.

MARGARET M. GINSTER, RN, AAS, BA, received two years nurses training at St. Conal's Hospital, Letterkenny, Ireland and one year at St. James Hospital, Portsmouth, England. She became a nurse after she won a six-year scholarship in order to become a schoolteacher in Ireland, but chose nursing instead. Influenced by cousins who were nurses in England, Margaret sailed from England to 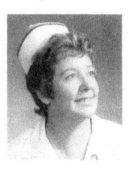 USA and held various nursing positions for six years before marrying.

Graduated from Saginaw Valley University with BA in sociology, 1986 and from Ferris State University School of Nursing (upper level), AAS in nursing, 1975. She has special training in psychiatric nursing and counseling; counseling in substance abuse, 1974, Traverse City State Hospital under supervision of Ferris State University School of Nursing; advanced first-aid CPR, 1974; In Service Training RN's pharmacology, 1976; Wayne State University, Oncology, Cancer Nursing, St. Mary's Hospital, 1977; nursing care of patient on ventilator, 1980; substance abuse services of Saginaw County, 1981; cardio vasular tech/meds cardiovascular diseases, 1987; and technical skills home care nursing, 1989.

Employment: Temporary Health Care Providers Inc., Midland, MI, 1978-80; Private duty homes and hospitals: St. Mary's, St. Luke's and Saginaw General; Staff Relief, Medical and Surgical Units, Bay Osteopathic Hospital; Med Nurse, Bay Osteopathic Hospital; Med Nurse, Geriatrics; Charge Nurse, supervising nurse's aides and LPNs; and part-time volunteer work for developmentally disabled, Saginaw County Association for Mentally Retarded Children, 1970.

Member of American Nurses Association, Michigan Nurses Association, District Nurses Association and Macomb Oakland Association for the Developmentally Disabled.

Widowed after 49 years of marriage to Saginaw attorney. She has five children (three are attorneys, one MBA and oldest son has cerebral palsy). Her husband had a stroke at age 58 and she gave nursing care to him for 15 years and is still involved with her oldest son who lives in group home. Presently semi-retired, she has five grandchildren, loves to travel, does volunteer work and visited Ireland after a 30 year absence.

FRANCES BEALL GIULIANI, RN,

MEd, decided she wanted to be a nurse after seeing movie, *Angels In White* (Florence Nightingale) while in elementary school.

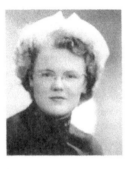

Professional Experience: Medical Record Review, Identification Infections, Sinai Hospital, Detroit, 1993; Telemetry Staff, Mt. Carmel Mercy Hospital, Detroit, 1990-91; Hospital Epidemiologist, developed and directed Hospital Infection Control Program at William Beaumont Hospital, Royal Oak, MI, 14 years; teacher of science and math., sec. public schools, Bloomfield Hills, MI, 3 years; assist. director of nursing, The Grace Hospital, Detroit, MI, 4 years; instructor of microbiology and chemistry, Sparrow School of Nursing Lansing, MI, 2 years; Labor and Del. Staff; Med/Surg. H.N., Sparrow Hospital, Lansing, MI.

Honors: RN, Boards of Nursing, Michigan, Indiana, Illinois; Michigan Secondary Provisional Teaching Certificate; Board Certified in Infection Control (CIC) 1984; Member APIC, American Nurses Association, MNA Expert Witness IC, MNA, AIDS-Speakers Bureau, Healthcare Risk Management Certificate, Amer. Inst. Medical Law, Inc. 1995; *Who's Who In American Nursing* 1984, 1986; Honor Society of Nursing, Sigma Theta Tau Int'l; contributor to *"89 Reasons To Be A Professional Nurse,"* published 1989; Board of Directors, MSU College Natural Science Alumni Association, 1990-96.

Education: Wayne State University, Detroit, MI; MEd, 1954; Michigan State University, BS, 1949; Mayo Clinic Association School of Nursing, Rochester, MN, Diploma of Nursing, 1946; Purdue University, IN; (undergraduate, 2 years).

Continuing Education: Amer. Inst. Med. Law, Healthcare Risk Management, 120 Hr.,

1995; U of Mich., Grad. Sch. Pub. Health, Biostatistics, 4 Grad. Cr. Hr., 1988; U of Minn., Grad. Sch. Pub. Health, 11 Grad. Cr. Hr., 1984, epidemiology of bacterial and viral diseases, Hospital Infection Control; U of Mich., Grad. Sch. Pub. Health, 11 Grad. Cr. Hr., 1973-75.

Conferences & Seminars: Assessment of Quality Medical Care/Quality Management, APIC-Detroit, 1991; Michigan Safety Conference, MIOSHA & MDPH, 1989; AIDS, Dr. Gallo, Hurley Hospital, 1989; Amer. Assoc. Med. Admin., 6 Hr. 1988; Assoc. Pract. Infect. Control (APIC), Annual Conf., 1973-83; Microbiological Aspect of Infection Control, Harvard Med. Sch., 30 Hr., 1978; Infections & Infection Control in Hospitals, U of Pittsburgh Sch. Med., 17 Hr., 1975; Legal Research & Writing I and II, Oakland University; 4 CEU, 1975; Surveillance, Prevention, and Control of Hospital Infections, CDC, 100 Hr., 1971.

Member Am. Nurs. Association, Healthcare Study Tour, Peoples' Republic China, 1979; Member of Healthcare I.C. Delegation to Chinese Med. Association and presented paper, 1986; Member Peace Study Group to Jordan, Isreal, Egypt, 1988 to Russia and Uzbekistan, 1990; American Red Cross, Nurse Volunteer, Northern California Disaster, 1989. She is now retired.

MARION GLENN, RN, born May 16,

1919 in Fowlerville, MI, the fourth child of seven. Early in life she became a very caring person by helping to care for her younger siblings. During her high school years she worked after school and Saturdays for a childless couple. She prepared dinner, served it and left the kitchen in order. On Saturdays,

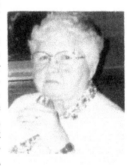

Marion did the baking and a more thorough cleaning of the kitchen. Marion graduated from high school in 1937.

Marion had hopes of someday being a nurse although the possibilities were remote. Much to her surprise and joy this couple offered to cover her expenses. Marion was accepted by the Bellevue Hospital School of Nursing in New York City for their nursing program. The help this couple gave relieved Marion of worry and made her time at Bellevue even more rewarding. She graduated in 1941.

During this time Marion met her future husband, Fredrick E. Decker, also a nurse in training at Mills School of Nursing at Bellevue Hospital. After graduation they were married and moved to Flushing, Long Island, NY. Soon after her husband was drafted to serve in WWII, Marion continued the work at

Queen's General Hospital in Flushing, NY, doing what she loved so much - Pediatrics. Illness of her mother-in-law caused Marion to move to Avoca, NY and she did industrial nursing at a factory in Hammondsport, NY. This little factory had grown from 15 employees to 400 during WWII and Marion commuted 25 miles to work. The fins, rudders and pedal assemblies did much to help in the war effort. Upon her husband's return they moved to New Hampshire where Frederick managed the Pharmacy at Laconia Hospital. During their stay in New Hampshire their son Glen Paul was born.

It was interesting that at Bellevue when children ate poorly, dessert was offered as an incentive. This usually helped. This plan did not work with the children from New York. Most were children of wealthy parents who sent their children to summer camps. Some parents did come, but it was not the norm. For these children dessert was no reward! They could care less!

Following a two-year stay in New Hampshire, the family decided to move to Jackson, MI, Marion's home state.

Her husband became an engineer on the New York Central Railroad and she returned to nursing. She worked at W.A. Foote Memorial Hospital for 25 years (five of them as staff nurse and 20 as head nurse of Pediatrics.

Marion has continued her interest in nursing and has had continuous registration in Michigan. This registration requires 25 credits each two years. It is a pleasure earning them and even though she is 84 years young she still feels she could help in an emergency.

Marion feels her life has been blessed by God. Even though there were difficult times, they seemed to make the good times even better. A wonderful husband and son and beautiful memories - what more could one ask?

DIANE DOMKE GODDEERIS, born

in Grosse Pointe, MI. She was recruited into nursing early because of nurses she met when hospitalized numerous times as a child. She received a nursing scholarship to the University of Michigan where she graduated with her BSN in 1977. Over the years, she has worked as a staff

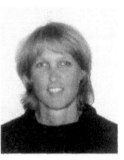

nurse and nursing instructor in her favorite area - Obstetrics. She is active with the Professional Employee's Council of Sparrow Hospital as a grievance and bargaining team member and currently is their vice-chairperson. Diane serves as Chapter 6's representative to the MNA Board of Directors and for the past two years, she has been on the editorial advisory board for *The American Nurse*. She was the recipient of the Economic and General Welfare Achievement Award in 2002. Diane resides in East Lansing, MI with her husband of 27 years and three children: Laura, Charles and Mary.

THOMAS F. GOODMAN, RN, born

Feb. 26, 1959, Muskegon, MI. Earned his BSN from Northern Michigan University in 1983. After graduation he was RN in the USAF until 1987; RN at Detroit Medical Center, 1987-88; RN at Hackley Hospital 1988 to present.

Thomas and his wife Diane have two children, Robyn and Mariel. Currently he is an RN in the emergency room at Hackley Hospital.

DELLA MAE MCGRAW GOODWIN,

RN, MSN, graduated from Paul Laurence Dunbar High School of Little Rock, AR, as

co-valedictorian, May 1950. Denied admission, for reasons of race, to mainstream institutions at Little Rock, Detroit and District of Columbia, Della entered Freedmen's Hospital Diploma School of Nursing

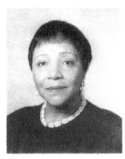

in DC in 1952. Freedmen's, established during the Civil War to serve fleeing and freed slaves, was for Della what it had been for her forebearers - a refuge from the artificial barriers imposed by racial injustice. Della graduated Summa Cum Laude in 1955.

Rounding out her formal education, Della earned BS (with distinction) and MS (US Public Health Service Fellow) degrees at Wayne State University in Detroit. She also completed post-graduate study in the history and philosophy of education.

By the late 60s and early 70s, Della's professional achievements had taken her to boards and commissions at the state level where she served on the Nurse Recruitment Committee of the Michigan League for Nursing. In this role she served on advisory panels of the Michigan Health Council, and provided testimony to the Michigan Department of Education, advocating for a "new" program in Wayne County, that would prepare the registered nurse to meet the needs of Detroit Central City hospitals.

Retained by Wayne County Community College as a consultant to start a Practical Nurse Program, she advocated for an Associate Degree Program to prepare the Registered Nurse. The mission was to serve an urban population that had been excluded from similar programs in the county for reasons of race, education, or jurisdiction; 10 existing programs failed to admit non-white applicants in significant numbers.

Della sought and secured community support for the program and garnered federal grants totaling $850,000 as start up funding. Attracting research funds, Della documented the admission, progression and graduation of students. *A Formula to Admit and Retain the Non-Traditional Student in Nursing* was published in 1975. This and subsequent publications, documented the characteristics predictive of success in nursing for the population served. A computerized admissions formula was implemented.

The first class was admitted on Sept. 14, 1972. By 1986, an estimated 3,360 applicants gained admission. Over a 14-year period more than 2,500 graduates completed the program and were eligible to write the licensing examination for Registered Nurses in Michigan. The average graduate was a 37-year-old black woman, married, with two or more dependents. A majority had been employed in area hospitals as Licensed Practical Nurses, Nurse Assistants and other entry-level workers; 55% were non-white and 10% were men. The program continues today in its 30th year.

Upon her retirement in 1986, The Board of Trustees of the College bestowed upon Della the title "Dean Emeritus." In October 2002, graduates celebrated the 30th year anniversary of the program. The Detroit City Council adopted a resolution extolling the contributions Della has made to the citizens of Michigan that will reach far into the future. She was inducted into the Michigan Women's Hall of Fame in 1997.

Della was the first recipient of the Bertha Lee Culp Human Rights Award of the Michigan Nurses Association, Commission on Human Rights, in 1985. She was active with the Detroit District Nurses' Association, Head Nurse, Nurse Administrator, and Nurse Educator units as she advanced in her career. She was appointed to the INPUT Board of Trustees in 1986; Della was nominated by MNA for a position on the Cabinet on Nursing Education of the American Nurses Association in 1984. Appointed by the ANA Board of Directors, she served 1984-86.

In 1974, the Michigan Nurses' Association nominated Della to serve on the Board of the federally designated, Comprehensive Health Planning Council of Southeastern Michigan. During her 10-year tenure on the board, she was elected president (1979-81). As president Della presided over proceedings that resulted in the development and implementation of the "Plan for Reduction of Excess Hospital Capacity." She gained stature as an advocate for vulnerable populations and engineered effective strategies to improve access to care for 4.5 million people in the seven county area.

SHARON L. TRAVIS-GOVAN, RN,

born June 22, 1966, Indianola, MS. She made Dean's List and earned her BSN from Eastern Michigan University in May 2004.

Assignments include travel agency RN

for five years; worked in 15 hospitals and private homes in following areas: rehab, spinal cord injury, telemetry, LTC, med/surg in five states.

She opened her own nursing agency in August 2002 to continue her practice as an independent RN contractor. She is a member of the Nurses Guild at her church, Northwest Unity Missionary Baptist Church, and is in the process of starting parish nursing there as well. Currently, RN to BSN completion program at EMU then on to University of Michigan to complete the FNP/MBA program.

Sharon, the fourth of six children, vacations about three times a year in Indianola, MS, where her parents, Joe and Mattie Lyions live.

LORRAINE WICKE GOWARD, born

in Owosso, MI, planned on entering nursing school upon graduation from high school in 1970. However, a

family health emergency, and later marriage and family sidelined those plans. She went on to work in the health field as a health technician and phlebotomist.

When her husband died suddenly in 1989,

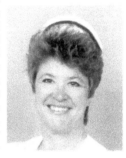

leaving her with three young children to rear, she once again entertained thoughts of becoming a nurse. When her youngest child entered second grade, she enrolled in Great Lakes College's Nursing Ladder Program in Midland, MI. (Great Lakes College later became Davenport University.) In 1997 Lorraine graduated second in her class from the first step of the ladder and obtained her practical nurse license. Her dream was finally realized the next year when she completed her associate degree in applied science and graduated with high honors. She obtained her license to practice as a registered nurse in September 1998.

She has worked as a charge nurse supervisor in the local nursing home and, most recently, as a psychiatric nurse in community mental health. She quickly became active in the local MNA staff council. She was elected chair in 2002. In 2003 she volunteered to act on the MNA's E&GW Nominating Committee. She actively encourages young people to explore nursing as a career, and has influenced several family members, friends and co-workers to enroll in nursing programs.

She remarried in 1999. She has one daughter, currently studying to become a nurse, two sons, and four stepsons. She and her husband Joe have eight grandchildren with two more on the way. She gives thanks and glory to her heavenly Father who has shown great mercy and love as he guides her throughout her life.

GAIL (FISHER) GRANNELL, RN, BSN, LPN, CHIP, earned LPN at Kirtland Community College in 1979; ADN at Lansing Community College in 1984; and BSN at Excelsior College in 1992. In 1997 she was featured in *Who's Who Among American Nurses.*

Assignments include staff RN, pediatrics, Sparrow Hospital for 23 years and one year as Med/Surg float. Healing touch practitioner, she works with balancing the personal energy field to bring into balance to enhance the healing process. She is MNA Chapter 6 president, E&GW cabinet secretary, volunteers at Healing Touch Center, Farmington Hills.

Divorced, she has elderly parents, four siblings, three nephews, one niece and four cats.

CONNIE L. GREENE, BSN, MSN, born at home in Monticello, IN. She became interested in pet care while just a toddler and later as a grade school student. One of her early essays was titled "My Home is a Zoo," She had considered vet medicine, but due to her own medical needs as a child with facial dog bites, she became aware of the office of their family physician and his nurse. Both the MD and the RN were true professionals who could handle the multitude needs of various patients. They were both active in the community and were considered positive and valued contributors to Monticello.

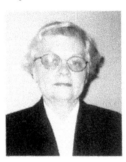

She started to consider nursing as a career goal in response to the office nurse (who by the way had assisted the MD to deliver her at her family's home) as a role model for what a nurse could be. She was also urged, especially by her father, to get a "sheep skin." — his way of saying graduate from college.

During her high school years a nurse recruiter from Indianapolis Methodist Hospital talked with their school's future nurses' club. They also talked with another local nurse who was one of the county health nurses.

She decided to attend the Methodist diploma program and later enrolled in Indiana University's extension program at Indianapolis where she attended many classes after receiving her nursing diploma.

Ultimately she earned three "sheep skins" and has enjoyed a very rewarding career as a medical-surgical nurse and educator, BSN, MSN (minor in education) from Indiana University and a PhD in Sociology (Family, Medical Organizations, Health Care Teams) with a minor in public administration from the Ohio State University.

She has been an active member of the Washtenaw/Livingston/Monroe, Chapter (Chapter 8) of the MNA since 1975. She has served as MNA and ANA delegate for several years. She is Past President and one of Chapter 8's Public Policy representatives to their Board.

She has enjoyed her work with MNA and especially the networking with MNA colleagues. Her motto, "I always get more from my MNA work than I give!"

DORIS M. GREENFIELD, born March 1, 1923, Hastings, MI. Graduated Hastings High School in 1940. She did not consider working outside the home until 1955. Her mother-in-law had a nursing home and she started working there, taking care of senior patients.

Barry County built in 1985 a medical facility, one of the first in Michigan. She started as a 3-11 shift nurse's

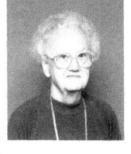

aide and was one of the first employees. She did patient care and medication under RN supervision. An in-service RN gave a 72 hour class and she (Mariom Sorby) suggested that Doris go back to school to be a nurse.

She earned her associate degree in nursing from Kellogg Community College in 1967. After graduation she continued working at the facility as a 3-11 supervisor, was advanced to day shift as assistant director of nursing until retiring in December 1985. Doris earned her bachelor's in health study from Western Michigan University in 1980.

Received Barry County Historical Society Award for Distinguished Service in the preservation of Barry County history and the PAT Award (Positive Action for Tomorrow) for extra ordinary service to the Red Cross for 20 years. She is a life member of Michigan Nurse Association.

Currently, she volunteers at Red Cross Blood Bank (20 years); Commission of Aged doing Blood Pressure Clinic; and to Thornapple Manor Facility for patient trips.

ARDITH GRIFFIN, RN, born Oct. 21, 1944, Lapeer, MI. Earned her associate degree at Mott College. Worked one year at Crittenton Hospital and from 1987-2003 at Lapeer Regional Hospital as RN. Currently, she is working in intensive care at Lapeer.

Ardith was delegate to convention and for

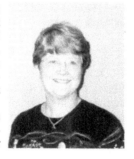

five years has been Chapter 4 Treasurer of Lapeer RN Staff Council.

Married 40 years to Ronald, and they have three daughters and three grandchildren.

JOAN GUY, BA, born Dec. 20, 1926, has diploma in nursing and BA. Assignments include college, staff office, head nurse (varied settings) and nursing administration (MNA).

She received Distinguished Service Award, Humanitarian Service Award, Sigma Theta Tau (Alpha Psi Chapter). Honorary trustee, ANF; NSNA and MSNA honorary memberships; Michigan Women's Commission and member of National Task Force on Credentialing in Nursing. She was elected secretary, ANA; ANA Consultant to NSNA and ANF vice chairperson and trustee.

Currently, she is active in local government (Zoning Board of Appeals and Planning Commission) and is an avid gardener and traveler.

JENNIFER H. MERRITT-HACKEL, RN, MS, CS, CDE, born July 29, 1958, Rochester, NY. Earned her BSN in 1980, UM; MSN in 1984, UM; and Specialist in Aging Certificate, 1984, Institute of Gerontology.

Assignments include UM Hospital Cardiac Unit, 1980-82; Rehab RN, 1982-84; Adult NP Planned Parenthood of

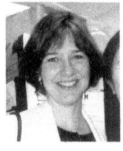

Mid-Michigan, 1984-85, gerontological nurse practitioner at UM-Turner Clinic, 1985 to present.

Received Emily Gleason Sargent Award (Community Health Nursing), Certified by American Nurses Credentialing Ctr., Gerontological Nurse Practitioner and Certified Diabetes Educator. Member of Sigma Theta Tau, Rho Chapter, American Geriatric Society, American Diabetes Association and American Academy of Nurse Practitioners.

She enjoys precepting students. Jennifer participated in research on older adults undertaking intensive insulin therapy for diabetes, 1986-96. Since 1989 she has run a diabetes support group at the clinic. She loves being a nurse practitioner in dynamic academic environment.

Jennifer had two daughters, Carolyn (14) and (Jaime) 16; she remarried in 2001 to Richard Hackel.

KATHLEEN HALLER, RN, born May 6, 1936, Eagle Bend, MN. Diploma in nursing, Rockford Memorial Hospital, Rockford, IL; BSN, Northern Illinois University, Dekalb, IL; MSN, Michigan State University, Lansing, MI.

Assignments as clinical instructor, obstetrics, Rockford Memorial Hospital in

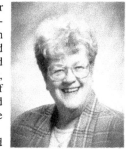

Illinois, director of staff development, Butterworth Hospital, Grand Rapids, MI, and clinical faculty, Kirkoff School of Nursing, Grand Valley State University.

Received honorable mention, Journal of Nursing Administration. Member of MNA, 1992-2004; Illinois Nurses Association, 1972-76; Sigma Theta Tau, Kappa Epsilon, Nursing Honor Society, 1992 to present; Congress on Nursing and Health Care Economics, MNA, 1998-99, chairman, Grand Rapids, Nursing Staff Development Coordinating Committee, 1982-83.

Kathleen and Christian have been married since 1958 and have three daughters: Anne Wildfong, Barbara Moser, Joyce Weise; and three granddaughters: Nicole, Christa and Amanda. Kathleen is retired and caring for husband with multiple myeloma.

JEAN Y. PATTON HALLEY, born June 14, 1932, Detroit, MI. Educated in Detroit Public Schools and graduated from Cass Tech High School in June 1951. Worked as licensed practical nurse from 1959-73. She graduated from Schoolcraft College in 1973 with an associate degree. Upon passing State Boards worked as an RN in general medicine, hemodialysis, and pediatrics at the city of Detroit Health Department until retirement Sept. 11, 1991 with 30 years of service.

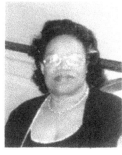

Post Retirement: Volunteer for the Arthritis Foundation of Southeastern Michigan, Healthy Living Project and helps with senior flu shots for city of Detroit. A member of Mayflower Congregational United Church of Christ, President of Detroit Public Health Nursing Alumnae, serves as secretary-treasurer of Michigan American Federal State County and Municipal Employees Council 25, City of Detroit Retirees Sub-Chapter 98, maintains membership in Michigan Nurses Association and a life member of NAACP.

Jean and husband Nathan are parents of Nathan III (md. Karen), Elijah (md. Cathi), Anthony F. Sr. (md. Maggie) and Mario P. (md. Kim).

She is currently taking lessons in duplicate bridge for fun, taking trips to interesting places and visiting great-grandchildren.

JONNIE M. PERRYMAN-HAMILTON, born in Tyler AL, the fourth of 10 children

who were always interesting in helping others. Her favorite childhood game was doctor. She decided to become a nurse when medical school was financially prohibited. Nursing became her love and passion. She graduated from Providence Hospital School of Nursing with a Diploma in 1973, received a certificate as a Pediatric Nurse Practitioner from University of Michigan in 1980, BSN and MSHA from the University of Detroit in 1985 and 1987.

She has worked in nursing at a variety of positions from staff nurse to director and has taught in several schools of nursing. She currently is practicing as a nurse practitioner in a school setting.

Jonnie has received many awards for her professional and civic accomplishments a few are 1987 Detroit Free Press, RN of the year, Search for Excellence Award, Berth Lee Culp Human Rights Award, Advanced Practice Nurse of the Year, Maternal Child Health Achievement Award, all from the Michigan Nurses Association (MNA). She also received the Advanced Practice Nurse of the Year Award from the National Black Nurses Association (NBNA), and the Special Achievement Award from Chi Eta Phi Sorority, Inc.(CEP).

She served MNA as a board member for eight years and an elected delegate to the ANA and MNA conventions since 1980. She has held leadership roles in other professional nursing organizations that include, NBNA, MBNA, NAPNAP and CEP. She is a member of Linwood Church of Christ in Detroit, MI was married, has three adult children, four grandchildren, and one great-granddaughter.

GAYLIA HANSON, Staff RN, Charge RN, born May 25, 1957, Plainwell, MI. Earned her ADN, Southwestern Michigan College, 1978 and BSN, University San Diego, 1983. Member of MNA, 1983 to present.

Assignments: 1978-79, Bronson, floor staff; 1979-80, Mercy, San Diego, MICU; 1981-83, house coordinator, charge RN, Neuro ICU; 1984 to present, staff RN and charge, Cardiovascular Lab, Borgess Medical Center, Kalamazoo, MI.

Gaylia and David have been married 20 years and have two children, Alex and Chelsey.

PHYLLIS J. HARPER, born May 26, 1934, Saginaw, MI. Staff nurse, Aleda E. Lutz VA Hospital, 1955-64; Public Health nurse, 1964-72 with city of Saginaw (merged with Saginaw County Dept. of Public Health in 1973); Senior Public Health Nurse 1981 to retirement in 2000.

She was named Employee of the Year (twice) and Nurse of the Year (once), received group award from Michigan Dept. of Public Health for copyrighted baby pamphlets they developed.

Activities include Board of Directors, Saginaw District Nurses Association, MNA Board of Directors (two year term), served

on MNA and E&GW Committee and board of directors, East Central District.

Chair person in 1966 when MNA and the city of Saginaw Public Health Nurse Staff Council signed the first ever union contract with the city of Saginaw. In 1973 the Saginaw County Public Health Nurses Staff Council signed with MNA the first contract for Public Health Nurses with the county of Saginaw.

Phyllis retired in 2000. Her husband is deceased. Oldest daughter is certified pediatric nurse practitioner and works in private practice; middle daughter is LPN at local nursing home and rehab center and youngest daughter is postal employee.

LYNNE HARRIS, born in Saginaw, MI. She attended the University of Michigan studying to become a teacher. Twelve years later, after marriage and the birth of four children, she received an associate degree in nursing from Henry Ford Community College.

Moving to Mesick, she was a staff nurse at Cadillac Mercy Hospital, nurse for Cadillac schools, teacher of health careers at the area vocational center, and on faculty at Northwestern Michigan College. She worked summers at Traverse City Osteopathic Hospital.

She has been active in MNA since graduation in 1972, holding elected positions in the Wexford-Missaukee and Northwest Districts as well as appointment to the MNA Board from the Northern Great Lakes Chapter.

She obtained her bachelor of science in nursing from the University of Michigan in 1979 and a master's degree in nursing from Wayne State University in 1985. In retirement, she serves on her local school board.

DEBRAH DEE HARTWICK, born Feb. 19, 1950, Bay City, MI. Earned her BSN at University of Michigan School of Nursing. Assignments include University of Michigan, Staff Nurse, Medical ICU Staff Nurse, Clinical Nurse I, II, III, and currently Clinical Nurse Supervisor, Mott Children's Hospital (U of M) which is a pediatric med/surg unit.

In 1994 she received Washtenaw-Livingston-Monroe Nurses Nurse of the Year Award, MNA E&GW Achievement Award in 1986, U of M Hospitals Nursing Executive Council Outstanding Contribution to Nursing Service Award, UMPNC Bargaining Team Data Group in 1994 and MNA Recognition of Service Award in 1993.

Debrah has held numerous MNA positions, board of directors, E&GW Commission, Bylaws Comm., ANA Delegate; Chapter 8 activities: board of directors, Nominating Comm., Bylaws Committee, MNA Delegate; UMPNC: officer, grievance rep. and bargaining team member.

Some of her memorable experiences include being MNA board member when they moved office; ANA Delegate when changed to a federation; UMPNC bargaining when they went on strike twice; ANA and MNA conventions.

DORIS H. HASAN, MNA CEAP Administrator, born in Massilon, AL. She was inspired by her science teacher to pursue nursing as career and earned her diploma of nursing at Hurley Hospital of Nursing in 1970; BSN, University of Michigan in 1977; MSN, Wayne State University in 1984.

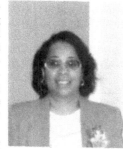

Doris had assignments as staff nurse, charge nurse on medical/surgical units, staff development instructor, director staff development and clinical development and clinical associate UM-F.

Awards include Nurse of the Year, GLSDNA and GFBNA Employee of the Month, Hurley Medical Center. Certified (ANCC) Nursing Administration and Nursing Continuing Education and Staff Development, American Heart Association BLS Instructor and Trainer.

She is a member of MNA CEAP, Healthcare Mentor through FACED, treasurer, UM-F Alumni Board of Directors, NBNA 2nd Vice President, MCC member Advisory Committee, ADN program and member Pi-Delta of Sigma Theta Tau.

Divorced, she has two daughters, two sons, and is a member of Grace Emmanuel Baptist Church and Nursing/Health Ministry.

JOANNE WENTA HATCHER, born in a huge three story house known as Caro Hospital. In her second grade autobiography she listed "nurse" as her future occupation.

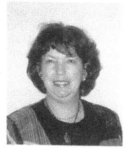

She received her diploma degree from Hurley Hospital School of Nursing in 1973. Soon afterwards, she began working at Lapeer County General Hospital. She has remained there for the past 31 years. She returned to school and graduated from U of M Flint in 1980 with a BSN degree, Cumma Sum Laude.

She married Vincent Hatcher in 1975 and they have two children. Nicole is 20 years old and a student at U of M Flint. Greg is a senior at Davison High School.

Joanne is a member of MNA and has been a delegate to the convention several times. She is a member of Chapter 4-Bay Central (served on their board for two years), Lapeer Staff Council (served as grievance representative for four years), and also Sigma Theta Tau International-Pi Delta Chapter.

She is a member of St. John's Catholic Church, school band boosters, and was on a community board to raise funds for a local skate park.

Her other interests center on her love of family, reading, and gardening.

DIANNE HAYWARD, RNC, MSN, WHNP, born in Detroit, MI at Art Center Hospital adjacent to the Wayne State University's (WSU) College of Nursing (CON). After spending 10 years at home with her children, she received her associate degree in accounting. For a few years she worked at *The Detroit News*. Thinking she wanted to become a pediatrician, she enrolled in pre-med at WSU in 1982. On the first day of class, luckily, she was unable to find a parking space so she went home.

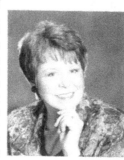

In 1983, she suffered a back injury and remained out of work for almost a year. During that year, she re-evaluated her life's direction. She obtained her ADN - RN in 1987. In 1990, she was the first student admitted to WSU's ADN to MSN program. She received her BSN in 1992 and her MSN in 1995. She has worked in med/surg, post-partum, pediatrics, NICU, L&D, and Antenatal Testing co managing high-risk pregnancies. She surprised everyone when she left Antenatal Testing with four years seniority to take a 7-week contract with WSU's CON. That was eight years ago and she has never regretted that decision. Prophetically, in high school, she was a member in both the Future Nurses' and Future Teachers' Clubs. Teaching nursing is her passion.

In 1996, she became certified as a Woman's Health Nurse Practitioner. She currently teaches full-time on a nine-month contract at WSU and adjunct at Oakland Community College, Highland Lakes Campus. She is a member of MNA, AWHONN, Sigma Theta Tau - Lambda, and MICNP.

She has two adult children and five grandchildren ranging from 2 years old to 18 years old. Her husband passed away four years ago, which not only impacted her life but also how she teaches and comforts others. Her article on grieving, *"Memories of a Loved One: From Caring Comes Comfort"* was published in AWHONN Lifelines, Volume 6, Issue 2, pp 179-180.

ANNETTE HELLER, RN, BSN, born July 11, 1960, Norway, MI. She earned her BSN at Medical College of Georgia; ADN and LPN at Bay de Noc Community College, Escanaba, MI.

Assignments include radiology RN, post CCRN working ICU open heart in Florida,

Georgia and as a traveling nurse in Trauma Burn at U of M, ICU in Mississippi and as a director of home care in Orlando, FL, worked ED, OB, OR, ICU and home call. Currently she is RN supervisor in radiology and radiation oncology nurse at Dickinson County Healthcare system in Iron Mountain, MI.

Annette received SCHS Nurse Excellence Award in 2003. Other activities include Alumnus CCRN, Certified in ACLS, PALS, Neonatal Resuscitation; speaker for radiology and radiation oncology; first radiology RN at Dickinson County Hospital and opened new open heart recovery unit in Naples, FL and opened radiation oncology at DCHS in November 2000.

Annette is married to Joseph, no children, but they have a golden retriever named Clancy.

BARBARA JEAN HENSICK, MSN, RN, CS, Clinical Nurse Specialist, initially joined the UMHS in 1979 as a staff nurse on a general medicine unit. After completing her BSN degree, she moved to the US Virgin Islands where she was employed in a local hospital's ICU and was also a cruise ship RN. She returned to UM and worked in the Diabetes Care Unit and as a float nurse on the adult med/surg units in between summers spent at SeaCamp in Big Pine Key, FL as the Resident Camp RN.

Returning again to UM for a third time Jean became the CNS for a medical unit in 1987 and has since remained in her current position.

In 1991 her vision initiated UM Nursing's Community Youth Program, sponsoring community youth education activities to enhance the image of nursing and promote nursing as a stimulating and rewarding career for both men and women. An array of health presentations and/or career development activities for preschool through high school age has been implemented within the Ann Arbor and surrounding schools. Other community events include the interactive nursing exhibit "Be A Nurse!" at the Ann Arbor Hands-on museum and "Yes! For Nurses" at the Ann Arbor District Library.

In recognition of her contributions she has received a number of awards for Excellence in Nursing Leadership from UH, MNA, ANA and Sigma Theta Tau.

For over 10 years Jean has been very active in the Michigan Nurses Association in numerous positions and is current board member.

KIMBERLY HICKEY was born in Columbus, OH, the eldest daughter with three younger siblings. Chemistry and literature were her favorite subjects in school. She decided to become a nurse during her junior high school year looking to it as a way to best utilize her skills.

She obtained her BS degree from Bowling Green State University, and her MSN from

Wayne State University in Primary Care Nursing with a minor in Gerontological Nursing in 1988. She is certified by the ANCC as an Adult Nurse Practitioner and as a Clinical Specialist in Gerontological Nursing.

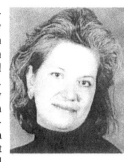

She received the Washtenaw-Livingston-Monroe Nurses Association Nurse of the Year award in 1995. She received the MNA Outstanding Gerontological Nurse award in 1995.

She served on her chapter board of directors, then was president of the Washtenaw-Livingston-Monroe Nurses Association 1990-92. She then served on the MNA Board of Directors 1992-96 representing gerontological nurses. From 1988-97, she assumed leadership roles in the MNA Nominations Committee, Reference Committee, Gerontological Practice Section, and Cabinet of Nursing Practice. Kimberly was the president of the Michigan Nurses Association 1997-99 during which time she represented the MNA on the Constituent Assembly and the State Nurses Association Labor Coalition. This was balanced with serving on the ANA Reference Committee 1997-2000.

Kimberly is one of only three nurses on the Ethnogeriatrics Committee of the American Geriatrics Society.

She has been a precinct delegate for the Republican Party since 1993. She has won election to serve on the Plymouth District Library Board of Trustees and is now in her third four-year term. She and her husband have had their names on the November ballot for the general election every other year since 1994.

CAROLYN HIETAMAKI, RN, became a nurse after a severe injury from a fall. She saw what it was like to be a patient and vowed to be a nurse who cared about the person in the bed.

She is a surgical floor staff RN and wound care RN at Marquette General Health System.

Carolyn received the E&GW Achievement Award. She is chair of her RN Staff Council, member and currently president of E&GW Cabinet, secretary of board of directors and board member of Michigan AFL-CIO.

She lives with her husband Robert in Gwinn, MI in the beautiful Upper Peninsula of Michigan.

BRIGID C. HINKLEY, BS, MA, born Sept. 18, 1927, Grand Traverse County. She is married and has five daughters and eight grandchildren. Worked as Public Health Nurse, OR Nurse in Mt. Pleasant; staff nurse and nurse practitioner, Central Michigan

University; Kent County Health Dept., Grand Rapids. She is currently retired.

ADA SUE HINSHAW, PhD, RN, is Professor and Dean of the School of Nursing at the University of Michigan. She was the first Director of the National Institute of Nursing Research at the National Institutes of Health. Her research interests are on 1) professionals who function in bureaucracies; job satisfaction, job stress, anticipated turnover and patient outcomes; 2) quality of patient care giving; and 3) instrument developed and testing of such measures as for patient satisfaction, job satisfaction of nurses and anticipated turnover of nursing staff.

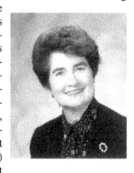

In addition, she has studied the use of ratio measurement techniques in building and testing the nurse and patient measures. Dr. Hinshaw is involved in a number of health policy activities; IOM committees such as the Work Environment for Nurses and Patient Safety and the Nursing Research Panel of the Parent Committee of Monitoring the Changing Needs for Biomedical and Behavioral Research Personnel. She has served on a number of national review committees and policy commissions; e.g., the Advisory Council for the Agency for Healthcare Research and Quality. She is past-president of the American Academy of Nursing, a member of the Institute of Medicine and a member of the IOM Governing Council. Dr. Hinshaw co-authored the first *Handbook for Clinical Nursing Research* and the text on *Magnet Hospitals Revisited: Attraction and Retention of Professional Nurses.* She has received numerous honors, awards and honorary degrees.

SHEILA HOAG, RN, born March 29, 1960, Grand Rapids, MI. She went to Lowell area schools and received her RN degree from Blodgett School of Nursing.

She worked at Blodgett Hospital after graduation and came to visiting Nurses Association where she has worked for the last 14 years. Recently she has joined the Hospice team.

Married for 24 years, Sheila and husband Kevin have three wonderful boys. She loves to work and help people out; she loves teaching patients and their family how to care for themselves or their loved ones.

MYRNA HOLLAND, born in South Bend, IN in 1940. She always planned to be a nurse and recalls admiring the nurse who gave her allergy shots. She read all the library books about nursing and from one learned about collegiate nursing education. In 1962 she

earned her BSN from Michigan State University and her MSN from Wayne State University in 1965.

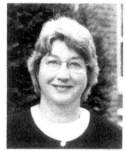

Her professional career includes staff nursing, teaching medical-surgical and psychiatric nursing, staff development, and nursing director. She retired as Director of Nursing Education and Performance Improvement, Providence Hospital in 2002.

Her service to MNA includes Detroit District Board, membership/marketing, Finance and Legislative Committees, MNA Board of Directors and MNA-PAC board. She served on the Restructuring Task Force and became the first president for the Southeast Chapter.

Accomplishments include Sigma Theta Tau, nursing administration certification, chairperson of Hospital Ethics Committee, a 40 year marriage, three successful children, and recognition by colleagues as a "Nurse's Nurse."

MILDRED OMAR HORODYNSKI, born in Baltimore, MD, and always wanted to be a nurse since she was 5 years old. Millie received her BSN from the University of Maryland in 1972, her MN from Wichita State University in 1978, and her PhD in Nursing from Wayne State University in 1989.

Dr. Horodynski is an associate professor at Michigan State University College of Nursing. She has lectured in Japan and taught in the Study Broad Program in Celaya, Mexico. She is actively engaged in research with a federally funded intervention study, Nutrition Education Aimed at Toddlers.

Dr. Horodynski received the inaugural Holmes Faculty Enrichment Award from MSU in 2001, and the Humanitarian Service Award from Alpha Psi Chapter, STTI. She is a Board member of Expectant Parents Organization and a childbirth educator.

She is married and has one married son and one daughter, who is also a nurse, just like her "mom."

KAREN HOVER, RN, born June 3, 1948, Paw Paw, MI. As a little girl she read a book about Nancy (nurse) and from that time on wanted to take care of people when they hurt or didn't feel good. Earned her associate degree from Jackson Community College and graduated as LPN in 1967.

She worked in Paw Paw,

Jackson, doctor's office and became an RN in 1983. Karen has worked seven years in pediatrics, 2-1/2 years in hemodialysis, south surgical specialties, float nurse and Observation Unit since opening of unit. Recently she accepted a position at Sparrow Mason Family Practice and will be starting the end of January.

Karen has worked on parish nurse committee while attending a local church, has helped in community service (time related with Sparrow Hospital). Married 35 years, she has two married children, Mark and Cyndi, and three grandchildren: Kelsie, Trevor and Dylan.

JUDITH I. HUBBEL, Staff Nurse, Nursing Supervisor, Nursing Consultant and Appeals Coordinator, born April 28, 1933, New Haven, CT. She earned her BS at Cornell University New York Hospital School of Nursing in 1956 and MS, University of Michigan in 1988.

Assignments include Washtenaw County PH Dept.; Livingston County PH Dept.; Hillcrest Regional Center; and Michigan Dept. of Mental Health.

Member of Sigma Theta Tau and MNA at district state level.

Judith and her husband Edward have two children, Herbert and Peter. She is currently retired.

HELEN FARRELL JAKEWAY, RN, BS, born June 25, 1924, Grand Rapids, MI. She was a member of Cadet Nurse Program while in nurses training. Earned RN at Mercy Central School of Nursing in 1945 and BS at Wayne State.

Employed at USVA Hospital, US Army Nurse, Macomb County Health Dept., school nurse in east Detroit for 18 years and nursing home for 20 years.

She has been a member of MNA for 50 years. Helen is now retired. She has one daughter and three grandchildren.

GAIL THOMPSON JEHL, LPN, born in Grand Rapids, MI and wanted to be a nurse from age four. She graduated from Grand Rapids Junior College as a licensed practical nurse in 1970. She attended and graduated from Ferris with her nursing degree in 1975. There she met and married Joe Jehl, and accomplished having four children in five years while continuing to work part-time.

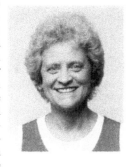

Her nursing jobs moved her to Port Huron, MI and Columbus, OH before settling down in Okemos, MI where she currently is employed as a staff nurse at Sparrow Hospital.

She became an advocate for practice issues. Starting in 1991, Gail served on the negotiation and bargaining teams for the Professional Employee's Council of Sparrow Hospital. She serves as her chapter representative to the Congress on Nursing Practice, a member of the MNA Board of Directors and has won the 2000 Economic and General Welfare Achievement Award.

CHERYL L. JOHNSON, BSN, born March 28, 1950, Dearborn, MI. When she was in high school, it seemed the most obvious job options for women were secretary, teacher, nurse. She saw them as sit down job, sit down job, stand up job, even though she had no idea what a nurse really did. She did get accepted into University of Michigan School of Nursing and upon graduation in 1972, was hired into a newly formed medical ICU at the University of Michigan (29 of her 32 years [and still working] have been spent in that unit).

In addition to that Cheryl has worked as a nurse at the University of Michigan football games, caring for spectators, and worked part time as a nursing instructor at both Eastern Michigan University as well as the University of Michigan Schools of Nursing. She has lectured for a company owned by Mt. Clemens General Hospital, presenting continuing education to nurses across the country.

Cheryl has served in various offices at her local, chapter, state and national nurses' associations. She is vice president of the American Federation of Labor by virtue of being President of the United American Nurses. She continues to enjoy what she does very much and advocates for herself, other nurses and patients through all of her work. Great work, good choice.

Awards include Med/Surg Nurse Achievement Award, 1990; Economic and General Welfare Achievement Award, 1995; Political Nurse Activist, 2001; Nurse Warrior Award, Chapter 8, 2002; and Mary-Ellen Patton, Staff Nurse Award, 2002.

EDNA G. JOHNSON, MSN, RN, C, born in South Carolina, became interested in health care after a neighbor encouraged her to become a nurse. She received a scholarship to attend Grady Memorial Hospital School of Nursing in Atlanta, GA. After graduation and passing the State Board Exam, she assumed a position with the South Carolina Department of Mental Health as nurse educator. She later married and moved to Hays, KS, where she worked in the emergency room and opened their first intensive care unit. She returned to South Carolina after having two children and began work at Moncrief Army Hospital at Fort Jackson, SC.

After eight years, she enrolled in the BSN completion program at the University of South Carolina and transferred to the Dorn Veterans Administration Hospital where she became the first African American Nursing Instructor. She completed requirements for the

BSN and MSN at the University of South Carolina. She worked at the Dorn VA Hospital for 10 years in many different roles and in 1986 was accepted in the Associate Chief, Nursing Service for Education Traineeship Program. After completion of this program in Richmond, VA, she assumed the position of Associate Chief, Nursing Service for Education in Alexandria, LA. In Louisiana, she was appointed by Governor Edwards to serve on Health Improvement Initiatives. While in Louisiana, she began work on a PhD in education at Grambling State University.

In 1992, she was appointed Associate Chief, Nursing Service for Education at the VA Hospital in Allen Park, MI. She retired from the John D. Dingal VA Hospital in Detroit in October 1997. In January, she began her present job, which she truly loves. She is the coordinator of the African American Hereditary Prostate Cancer Study at Wayne State University School of Medicine. She is also a part-time faculty member at Wayne County Community College District and the University of Phoenix-Michigan Campus. She recently enrolled in Capella University to complete the PhD in education.

She is a member of New Hope Missionary Baptist Church in Southfield, MI. She is a member of the American Nurses Association and Chi Eta Phi Sorority. She is divorced with three adult children, all in health care careers.

JANINE JOHNSON, Staff Nurse, RN, born June 10, 1962, Burbank, CA. Graduated Mott Community College as ADN, high honors.

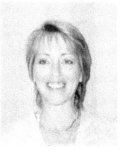

Employed at McKenzie Memorial Hospital (Med/Surg/ER); William Beaumont Hospital, telemetry; and currently RN, staff nurse in PACU at Lapeer Regional Hospital.

Married 20 years, she has three children and one grandchild. She is a member of MNA.

LOLA JOHNSON, RN, BSN, became interested in nursing while working at Dickinson County Hospital as a housekeeper. She entered Bay de Noc Community College Practical Nurse Program at the age of 37, and began practice in 1981. She became a RN after earning an associate degree in nursing from BDNCC in 1985,

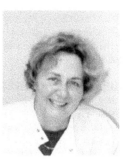

followed by a BSN from Northern Michigan University in 1990.

She received the hospital's Excellence in Nursing Award and was chosen by her peers as Employee of the Month.

Active at the district and chapter level, she currently sits on the Congress on Nursing Healthcare and Economics. She is vice-chair of the DCHS Staff Council, and has served on the Bargaining Committee for 13 years.

Having retired from DCHS as dialysis supervisor, she currently holds an irregular status, averaging two days per week. She remains an active member of Our Saviour's Lutheran Church.

Lola lives in Kingsford with her husband of 44 years, surrounded and blessed by children and grandchildren.

LAURA IRENE KAUFMAN, RNC NP,
born July 2, 1961, Ann Arbor, MI. Earned her BSN, Eastern Michigan University in 1985 and MS, University of Michigan Primary Care Program, Community Health Division in 1989.

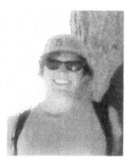

Assignments include provider primary care and podiatry care to the geriatric population in the clinic as well as several outreach locations in the community.

Awards include ANCC Certification as adult NP, 1989-present; Certificate of Appreciation Award for contribution to the educational experiences of nursing students for precepting nurse practitioner students 1996-present,

Laura gives talks to the community on aging changes. She is a member of Sigma Theta Tau, National Conference of Gerontological Nurse Practitioners.

Her most memorable experiences involve helping her patients heal, whether it be physical, emotional or spiritual; the relationships formed with them as a result of that bond are mutually satisfying.

Married 15 years, Laura and her husband enjoy growing organic fruits and vegetables, traveling and playing with their four dogs.

Today, she is continuing to learn and grow in caring for her geriatric patients and will be starting a new outreach clinic at University Commons, a community where retired faculty and staff live. She would like to be able to create a "wellness center" promoting healthy lifestyles in a holistic manner. It is a new and exciting opportunity for her. She is committed to not just surviving but thriving as a nurse practitioner.

DIANE M. KENNEDY, RN, born Dec.
27, 1957, Marlette, MI. Participated in Diploma Program at Hurley Hospital, then

worked as RN at Lapeer Regional Hospital ICU-CCUU on all floors including ER and PCU.

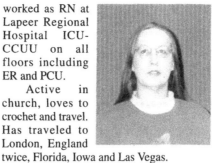

Active in church, loves to crochet and travel. Has traveled to London, England twice, Florida, Iowa and Las Vegas.

Currently working relief position, picking shifts mostly on midnight's. Diane and her husband Don have two children, both in college.

BARBARA KENNISON, PhD, RN, born
June 9, 1938, near Kalamazoo, MI. Attended Nazareth College at Kalamazoo for bachelor's, University of Washington in Seattle for master's, and University of Michigan for doctorate, clinical nursing research.

Assignments include lecturer, School of Nursing, U of M; asst. professor, psychiatric and community health nursing, Loyola University of Chicago; clinical director, Mental Health Services and director for clinical research, Michigan Home Health Care; private practice, individual and family therapy. Currently she is psychotherapist in private practice in Traverse City, MI.

Awards Include Who's Who Among American University, College Students, Professional Nurse Traineeship, American Journal Nursing Scholar, National Institute of Mental Health Education Grant Award.

Current member of American College of Forensic Examiners; Tri-County Coalition for the Prevention of Child Abuse and Neglect; Michigan Dept. Public Health Provider Institutional Care (Alzheimer's disease and related disorders task force); Michigan St. Medical Society AIDS Task Force; vice president of Michigan Professional Society on the Abuse of Children. Special interest is taking groups each year to Guatemala – San Andres to be with the Mayan people whose lives have been scarred by years of violence and destruction, leaving much sorrow and grief.

Barbara is also a member of the religious congregation of the Sisters of St. Joseph whose primary works are the education (of women and children), care of the sick and helping the poor.

LOIS AUSTIN KERR, RN, born Aug. 31,
1936, Pontiac, MI. Received her diploma from Henry Ford Hospital, Detroit, MI. Assignments include head nurse at Henry Ford Hospital, Detroit, MI; clinical nurse coordinator, William Beaumont Hospital, Royal Oak, MI; nurse manager, Michigan Masonic Home, Alma, MI.

Awards include 2003 Meijer Spirit of Volunteerism Recognition Award presented by United Way of Isabella County's Volunteer Center.

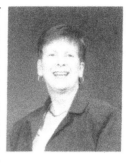

Member of MNA since 1958, she has attended MNA conventions and ANA conventions. She was delegate to MNA Convention twice and once to ANA Convention in Washington, D.C. Through Presbytery of Lake Huron, she was member of Committee for Migrant Health Fairs, and has planned and participated in fairs for past 12 years.

Retired, but still volunteers at Adult Day Program. She is a board member of Rosebush Interfaith Retirement Corp. and local Soup Kitchen.

MARY B. KILLEEN, BSN, MSN, PhD,
her background extends over 40 years of experience in the service and education settings.

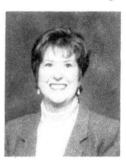

As noted by her credentials (CNAA, BC), she is certified in nursing administration. Advanced through ANCC. Her diploma is from Providence Hospital School of Nursing and her BSN, MSN (Advanced Maternity Nursing), and PHD degrees are from Wayne Statue University College of Nursing.

Nursing is her passion and her research role makes all the other work involved even more exciting. Her philosophy of nursing is based on Imogene King. She believes nursing is being alive with people. Her object of nursing care has shifted from the patient to the students that she teaches! When she was an administrator, the nursing staff were her "Patients." She is involved at the local, state, and national levels in the American Nurses Association with a focus on political action and health policy.

DEBORAH KNECHT, born in Illinois
but moved to Lapeer, MI as a child and has lived there since then. Her mother always told her she was going to be a nurse so when she graduated from high school, she went to Flint Jr. College (now Mott Community College) on a scholarship for their Associate's Degree Nursing Program. She was part of the last class to complete the program in two years.

Initially she worked at Flint Osteopathic Hospital in the Pediatrics Dept. In 1975 she went to Lapeer Regional Hospital and except for a four year period when she worked in a cardiologist's office, has been at LRH. At LRH she worked initially in ICU/CCU then in the OR. She was one of the first three nurses to become a BCLS instructor in 1977 and certified many of the LRH staff. She has also been ACLS certified since 1982. In 2001 she completed her certification for First Assist.

She has been married 31 years to Lewis and has two grown daughters, Erin and Andrea. Both daughters are married and are elementary teachers. She has one grandson, Alex. The element of nursing she loves most is the flexibility it offered her to rear two great daughters.

LINDA KRAUSE, Staff Nurse, RN, born Oct. 12, 1945. Earned her diploma RN, Grace Hospital School of Nursing in 1966. Employed in Recovery Room, Grace Hospital in Detroit.

Active in ASPAN and Staff Council. She is currently staff nurse, PACU, Cheboygan Memorial Hospital.

Linda and her husband John have two grown children, Dawn and Tim, and one grandchild.

LIZ YOUNG KRAUSE, MSN, BSN, RN, born 1925 in Sparks, GA. She entered nursing at J.H. Hospital because of a professor at Cumberland College, Williamsburg, KY, where she got her AD in 1945. Earned her BSN at J.H. Hospital in 1948 and MSN at Wayne State University in 1980. Research Practicum done under Virginia Cleland, College of Nursing, Wayne State University in 1979.

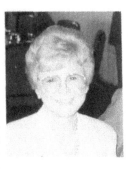

Employment: John Hopkins Hospital, Baltimore, MD, 1948-49; Edward W. Sparrow Hospital, Lansing, MI, 1949-53; Allegan General Hospital, Allegan, MI; Allegan County Health Dept., 1966-85, as public health nurse, asst. dir. of nursing and promoted to director of nursing in 1980; American Red Cross, Kalamazoo, MI Chapter as coordinator of Geriatric Health Screening Clinics, 1986-87; clinical instructor at Ferris State University, Big Rapids, MI, 1986-88 and at Hope-Calvin College, Holland, MI, 1986-90; Pullman Health Center, Pullman, MI, 1990-95, outreach nurse, Michigan Maternal Support Services and screening infants; VNA, Kalamazoo, MI, 1994-97, Early Maternal Discharge Program; VNA, Grand Rapids, MI, 1996-99, Early Maternal Discharge Program.

Liz served in leadership capacities for numerous professional organizations and community service groups.

She has three children: Robert, Konrad and Karen, and nine grandchildren (two grandson at West Point Military Academy).

JUDITH E. (RINN) (SMITH) KULKA, born in Saginaw, MI in 1940, reared in Midland, MI and graduated high school in 1958. She became interested in exploring nursing as a career as a result of a junior high school career exploration project. Her desire to combine science, psychology, college and nursing school led to attending Michigan State University, graduating in 1962 with a BSN, one of 16 graduates from an initial class of 100. Part of impetus for a career in nursing was recognizing the job market good for nurses wherever one might locate.

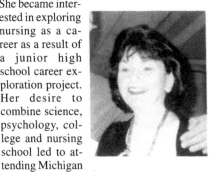

First nursing employment at E.W. Sparrow Hospital, Lansing, MI, medical/rehab unit, in 1962. Major portion of nursing career in public health nursing, as staff nurse and supervisor.

Earned master's degree in family studies (MSU) with a minor in supervision in 1981.

President of MSU College of Nursing Alumni Association 1973-78; one term as MNA Chapter 6 rep to Legislative Committee, two terms as Chapter 2 rep to CE Provider Unit (after retirement).

Married to Jerry for 24 years, she has a daughter Lisa in St. Louis, MO; adopted son Mark in Grand Ledge, MI; and stepson Don in Westland, MI.

Retired in 1996 from Ingham County Health Department after 22-3/4 consecutive years to northwest Michigan on Grand Traverse Bay. Retirement activities include quilting, bridge, travel, UFO Field Investigator for MUFON, hosting friends and relatives (initially some B&B guests too), and winter vacations in Sedona, AZ.

PAMELA G. LATIMORE, born in Detroit, MI, and became interested in nursing as a young girl. Her interest increased after becoming active in the Future Nurses' Club in high school.

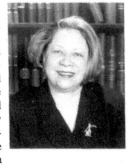

She received an associate degree in applied arts and science from Highland Park Community College and obtained her license to practice as a Registered Nurse. The early years of her nursing career were spent at Detroit Receiving Hospital. She held several different positions at Receiving including Head Nurse.

She obtained a bachelor of science

degree from Mercy College in 1979 and a master of arts in teaching degree from Wayne State University in 2000. She is currently employed by the Detroit Public School System.

She is a member of the Board of Directors of Hartford Memorial Baptist Church's Agape House. She is a volunteer speaker for the Karmanos Cancer Institute. She also serves as a site coordinator for Project Healthy Living.

She is a life member of Chi Eta Phi Professional Nurses' Sorority, Inc. She is also a member of Delta Sigma Theta Sorority, Inc.

She is a member of Hartford Memorial Baptist Church. She is married and the mother of two sons.

KATHLEEN MARIE LAW, LPN, LPN Team Leader, Staff RN, Clinical Leader CNI, II, III, born Sept. 5, 1952, Detroit, MI. Attended Shapero School of Practical Nursing at Sinai Hospital of Detroit (1971); Schoolcraft College for ADN (1984); Madonna University for BSN (1993); and University of Phoenix for MSN (1978).

Assignments: 1971-72, Sinai Hospital, Detroit; 1972-73, Killeen Nursing Home, Killeen, TX; 1976-77, U.S. Army Hospital, Berlin, Germany; 1977-78, Memorial Hospital, Manhattan, KS; 1979-80, St. Francis Hospital, Topeka, KS; 1980-93, Sinai Hospital, Detroit, MI; 1993-94, Home Health Plus; 1994-present, Providence Hospital, Southfield, MI.

Awards include Breakthrough to Nursing Award, Michigan Nurses Student Association, 1993 and *Who's Who in American Colleges and Universities,* 1992. She is certified in Ambulatory Women's Health Care, NCC, Madonna University Nursing Student Association, 1992-93 (vice president); Michigan Delegate to NSNA Convention in 1992; research, Women's awareness of gender differences in heart disease, 1999.

Other activities include Sigma Theta Tau International Honor Society of Nursing; Kappa Iota Chapter, Madonna University, 1993; RTS Bereavement Training in Pregnancy Loss and Newborn death, 1991; Kappa Gamma PI, National Catholic College Graduate Honor Society, 1993 to present.

Kathleen and Paul married in 1972; they have two sons, Jason and Joshua; and three grandchildren: Allison, Erin and CJ. Kathleen is currently care coordinator at Providence Hospital in Southfield, MI.

DEANNA MICHELLE LEMORIE, RN, born May 12, 1973, K.I. Sawyer AFB, MI, earned associate degree from Henry Ford Community College in May 2001 and currently working on BSN from Oakland University with intended date of graduation in December 2004.

Employed as RN, Henry Ford Hospital, 2001-02; RN, U of M Hospital on the orthopedic/trauma floor, 2002-present.

She is a member of MNA and NAON.

OPAL PATRICIA LESSE, BSN, MSN, APRN, FNP-C, born April 1, 1949, Coeburn, VA. She was influenced to be a nurse by her great-grand-mother Mary and great-aunt Dora, mountain medicine women, who cared for people with roots and herbs.

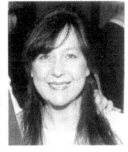

Attended Washtenaw Community College, LPN, 1978 Honors and ADN, 1983 Honors; U of M, BSN Cum Laude; Michigan State University, MSN, APRN, FNP.

Received U of M Team Leader Award, 1998, 1999 and 2002; Michigan Nurses Association "Nurse of the Year" in 2000; and Michigan State University Outstanding Alumni Award in 2002.

She was President Chapter 8 MNA, 2001-03; Vice President Chapter 8, 1999-2001; Delegate 1990-continued; Nominating Committee, 1995-99; adjunct professor, Eastern Michigan University; published Urology Inpatient Protocols/Research papers and U of M Speakers Bureau.

Active in Sigma Theta Tau, U of M Speakers Bureau and she is a volunteer NP for Hope Medical Clinic. Currently she is a nurse practitioner for the Urology Dept., U of M Health System.

Opal is the mother of five children and grandmother of seven.

ELSIE LETT, MSN, RN, born in Alexander City, AL became interested in nursing when she was 5 years old. She decided to become a RN after marrying and rearing one son. She received a Certificate in LPN shortly after completing high school. Years later, she returned to Wayne County Community College, obtaining an ADN in 1996, BSN from Eastern Michigan University and her MSN from the University of Phoenix (Southfield Campus) in 1998.

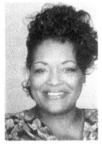

Elsie has been awarded numerous awards to include the MNA Award of Excellence in Nursing Practice, was recognized by Oakland University as a finalist for the Nightingale Award in the category of Education. She was nominated for the Robert Wood Johnson Health Policy Fellowship in 2000-01. She remains active in the nursing profession as adjunct faculty and mentor of nursing students while utilizing critical thinking, new knowledge and ideas to impact quality of life for Michiganians.

TARA LEIGH LINDLEY, RN, born Oct. 20, 1979, St. Lawrence Hospital. Earned her associates degree at Lansing Community College in December 2001. Also, laser certified.

Works as operating nurse at Sparrow Hospital. She is single and always has an eye looking out for Mr. Right.

JANICE LOCKE, BSN, NP, CNS, born in Detroit, MI, Janice always wanted to be a nurse. She received her BSN from MSU in 1981 and worked at Providence Hospital as a staff nurse and in staff development. In 1988, she returned to school in the Graduate Nursing Program at U of M.

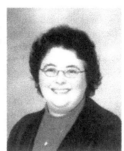

She received her master's degree in gerontological nursing in 1990 and went on to work at Glacier Hills Nursing Center in Ann Arbor - first as ADON and later as a Nurse Practitioner for U of M. Since 1997, Janice has worked in Senior Health Services, St. Joseph Mercy Hospital as a nurse practitioner. She is certified by ANCC as both an NP and CNS. She specializes in long-term care, urinary incontinence, wound management, advanced nursing practice issues and enjoys speaking on these topics.

In 2000, she was honored as Nurse of the Year by Chapter 8 of MNA.

TERRY LOGAN, LPN, RN, BSN, was born in Kingstreet, SC, and became interested in nursing as a child. Her mother is a nurse, She started in healthcare as a housekeeper, became a medical assistant, then attended the School of Practical Nursing in Detroit and became a LPN. She then went on to WCC and became a RN. She completed her BSN through Regents College.

She currently works as a nurse in outpatient gastroenterology at UMHS. She was the UMHS employee of the month in March 1996. She became a member of MNA in 1993 and served as a delegate from Chapter 8. Terry is well known to MNA and Chapter 8 members due to her advocacy work for safe needle legislation. She received the Nurse Warrior Award from Chapter 8 in June 2000 and the MNA Nurse Hero Award in October 2000.

Terry lives in Ann Arbor with her husband Melvin.

ORPHA R. (MATTSON) LOHMANN, RN, BSN, Clinical Instructor, Head Nurse, Charge Nurse, born Dec. 4, 1926 in North Dakota. Graduated high school in 1944; U.S. Cadet Nurse Corps, School of Nursing, Grand Forks, ND, 1944-47; BS, WSU, 1948-51.

She worked in obstetrics for about 25 years, was clinical instructor, OB and nursing, 1952-55; medical professional pool,

1967-72; charge nurse, relief night duty, Cottage Hospital, Grosse Pointe, MI, 1954-55 and was chairman of Economic Committee, NDS NA.

Activity: Alpha Theta Sigma, WSU, Detroit, MI; Beta Sigma Phi, National League of Nursing, North Dakota, 1952-54.

Married Peter Lohmann in February 1961 and has three grown children: Edward, Peter and Carlena. Orpha retired in 1990 and she did some home nursing until her health failed and prevented her from working.

ALICE LORENZ, grew up on a farm near Seward, NE. Maybe it was the farm experience that led Alice and her three sisters to all be nurses. She graduated from Lincoln General Hospital and worked as staff nurse, nurse manager and clinical instructor before moving to Michigan in 1973.

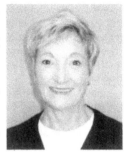

She moved with her husband, John, to Flint, MI when he accepted a position at GMI (now Kettering University). She worked for 28 years at Hurley as instructor, assistant director, Director of the School of Nursing, and Director of Education before retiring from Hurley in 2001. She is currently working at the UM-F/Hurley BSN program.

She is a member of the Board of Directors of the MLN and has served in multiple roles at MNA.

She has BS in health education from the University of Nebraska (1973) and MSN from Wayne State University (1982). She and her husband have one son.

JOYCE LOSEN, Data Entry, Membership Specialist, born Aug. 15, 1962, Alma, MI. An MNA staff member since 1991, Joyce works with member records, mainly those that do not involve bargaining units. Her responsibilities include coordinating monthly electronic dues payments, monthly credit cards, posting dues payments for members who pay on an annual basis, inputting members' address changes, and revising the association's leadership directory. She also processes the results of the yearly membership survey; handles recruitment and retention mailings and all mailings to students; and takes care of all registrations for the MNA's annual convention, Nurses Impact, and Leadership Planning Retreat.

Joyce attended Baker, Davenport and Lansing Community Colleges.

Her accomplishment was getting all three of her daughters through high school and into college as a single mom.

Married for three years and added two step-children to family. She has four grandchildren.

CARROLL A. LUTZ, a lifetime member, was MNA Membership Coordinator from 1977-79. She has held many offices in different districts and has been a member of several MNA Committees and the Congress on Public Policy.

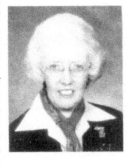

A graduate of St. Joseph Hospital School of Nursing in Hancock, MI and Marquette University College of Nursing in Milwaukee, she served as a staff nurse for the Veterans Administration and as a lieutenant in the U.S. Army. She taught at Bronson Hospital School of Nursing in Kalamazoo, Hurley Hospital School of Nursing in Flint, and retired from Jackson Community College in Jackson, MI.

She received the Mary M. Roberts Fellowship from the AJN and the AJN-MNA Excellence in Writing Award. She earned a master of arts in communication from Michigan State University. A book she co-authored, *Nutrition and Diet Therapy,* published by F. A. Davis, is going into the 4th edition.

MARILYNN JUFFERMANS MAGOON, born May 22, 1934 in Benton Harbor, MI. At the age of 5, she became interested in nursing. She graduated from the University of Michigan in 1956 with a BSN. She was a member of the first four-year nursing program at the university. She received a master of arts in education from the University of Michigan in May 1980.

She has worked as a head nurse, staff nurse, public health nurse and high school teacher in health occupations. She has served the University of Michigan and the Ann Arbor community in the following capacities: Henderson House Governing Board, Alumnae Council Governing Board, Medical Center Governing Board. She is presently an academy member of the Nursing Alumni Governing Board, serving on the Awards and Scholarship Committee. She is a member of the Margaret Waterman Alumnae Group, served as its president and organized the Town Hall series, which has raised $400,000 for scholarships awarded to undergraduate women at The University of Michigan. For her university work she has received a "Distinguished Service Citation" from the Alumnae Council Governing Board. She is a member of the Ann Arbor Thrift Shop, President 1999-2000.

She is a member of Washtenaw-Livingston-Monroe Chapter 8 of the MNA serving as delegate to MNA 1989-98. She received the Chapter 8 Hall of Fame Award in 1999, served as president 1996-98. She is a member of Sigma Theta Tau, Rho Chapter.

She is married to Dr. Duncan J.J. Magoon, a psychiatrist. She has reared four children: Duncan, Cameron, Molly and Jennifer, all graduates of The University of Michigan. She has five grandchildren. She continues to volunteer in the community, most recently at Hope Clinic in Ypsilanti, MI. She mentors University of Michigan freshman student nurses as they are doing their community service at the Ann Arbor Thrift Shop. She is grateful for her education and training. Some of her special mentors are Margo Barron, Norma Kirkconnell Marshall, and Hazel Avery.

She collects Blue Ridge Pottery and other antiques and enjoys bird watching.

MARIE (MELLON) MALONE, RN, BSN, CHPN (Certified Hospice and Palliative Nurse), born Aug. 28, 1939, Grant, MI. Earned Diploma RN in 1961, Blodgett Memorial Hospital School of Nursing, Grand Rapids, MI, and her BSN at Ferris State University, Big Rapids, MI, in 1990. Marie received the Nellie McCarty Scholarship.

Assignments: worked as staff and head nurse in ICU at Blodgett Memorial Hospital in Grand Rapids; staff and head nurse at Grant Community Hospital; clinical instructor LPN students, Muskegon Community College and instructor at local Nurse Aide Program. Since 1989 she has been clinical supervisor, Hospice of Michigan at Fremont, MI.

Marie started as nurse aide while sophomore in high school in 1956 in small local community hospital in Grant, MI. Memorable experiences include witnessing her first birth; and being clown "Nurse Raggedy Ann" to help cheer people.

Married 36 years, she has one biological son, two adopted older children and one grandchild.

SHERRI MANGAN, born May 5, 1958 and reared in northeastern Wisconsin. She graduated in 1982, Cardinal Stritch University in Milwaukee, WI, and began her career at Mount Sinai in Oncology/Hospice.

Moved near upper Michigan border in 1983 and began working at Dickinson County Hospital on surgical unit. Transferred to OR/PACU in 1986 and remains today.

Received CNOR in 1992, Nurse Excellence in 1999, and is chairperson of their Staff Council.

Sherri is married with three children – one of whom is in BSN Program at University of Wisconsin.

BARBARA MANN, RN, BSN, born Feb. 27, 1952, Valparaiso, IN. Graduated DePauw University School of Nursing in 1974 and passed boards the first try. In 1981 she was honored to give commencement address to her graduating seniors at Butterworth Hospital School of Nursing.

Assignments: 1974-75, Methodist Hospital, Indiapolis, IN; 1975-76 Ingham Memorial Hospital, Lansing, MI; 1976-81, instructor at Butterworth School of Nursing; 1982-84, ICU float RN, Butterworth Hospital School of Nursing, Grand Rapids, MI; 2003, Admissions RN, Hospice of Holland Home, Grand Rapids, MI

Other activities: 1999 - Certified Parish Nurse. She always knew she would be a nurse. Nursing is her soul and a natural way to share the grace that God floods upon her. She recently re-entered nursing after rearing her children and is currently Admissions RN at Hospice of Holland Home, Grand Rapids, MI.

PATRICIA MARKOWICZ, MSN, RN, born 1953 in Detroit, MI. 1976: graduated with high honors, cum laude, from Wayne State University's College of Nursing. Employed by Visiting Nurses' Association for Metropolitan Detroit. Been a member of Michigan Nurses' Association since 1976. Active in labor negotiations while at the VNA, and has

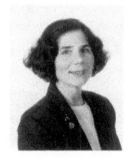

worked full-time in the field of nursing since then, mostly in the area of Community Health. She has traveled for fun throughout the USA and Canada by motorcycle with husband Mark Wiley these past 30 yrs.

1982: Married Mark. Moved to Saginaw area to become "ice cream barons" by opening a brand new Baskin-Robbins Ice Cream Franchise. Began work as a public health nurse for the County of Saginaw. Soon promoted to supervisory positions.

1990: Became first graduate of the Master's of Science in Nursing Program, administrative track from Saginaw Valley State University. Graduated with highest honors, summa cum laude.

1995: Became a nationally-certified motorcycle safety instructor. Teaches classes at Delta and Mott Community Colleges with Mark, who's been a motorcycle safety instructor since 1980.

Obtained current position as Associate Dean of Health Sciences Program at Mott Community College in Flint, MI. Demanding position, but always interesting, challenging, and holds much variety.

NORMA K. MARSHALL, PhD, was born Jan. 20, 1926 in Shepherd, MI and moved to Lansing, MI where she attended school and graduated from Lansing Eastern

High School in January 1944.

During the summer of 1943, she was employed as a nurse-aide at the Edward W. Sparrow Hospital. The nurses with whom she worked that summer were influential in her decision to apply for the nursing program there. The school, also, had an excellent reputation and selective admissions.

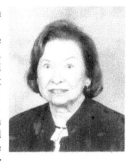

Norma graduated in 1947 from Sparrow's School of Nursing and while attending Michigan State University, she was an instructor in the nursing arts curriculum from 1947-51. She applied for admission to BSN program for Registered Nurses at Western Reserve University and earned her baccalaureate degree in 1952 and remained for three more semesters for the master of science degree in 1953. She earned a MA and a PhD in 1981 and 1985 from the Administration in Higher Education Program at the University of Michigan.

In the fall of 1953, Norma accepted a position at the University of Michigan as an assistant professor in charge of the Nursing Arts Program. She was promoted to associate professor with tenure in 1960 and to the rank of professor with tenure in 1972.

Positions held included head of an area of instruction, assistant dean for undergraduate studies, director of RN studies, Assistant Dean for Academic Affairs, Interim Dean of Nursing and Professor Emeritus of Nursing.

Professional activities include member and chair of the Washtenaw County Board of Health and Environmental Appeals, member and vice-chairperson of the Ann Arbor Township Planning Commission, member of the board of directors of the Michigan League for Nursing, member of Executive Committee of the Division of Education, Michigan Nurses Association, member of MCANE, Michigan Coalition on Articulation of Nursing Education (MNA), President of the Washtenaw, Livingston and Monroe District Nurses Association.

Awarded the MLN citation for "Outstanding Contributions for Improved Health Care in Michigan;" The UM Medical Center Award in recognition of "Service as a leader of the School of Nursing and for Contributions to the Improvement of Nursing Education." Recognition Award from Rho Chapter, Sigma Theta Tau for "Major Contributions to Nursing."

Member and Elder of First Presbyterian Church, Ann Arbor, MI. Norma is married to Claude J. Marshall and they have a daughter, Anne Harrell (William) and a grandson, John Marshall Harrell, all living in the Ann Arbor area.

DONNA J. MARTIN, RN, Staff Nurse, Charge Nurse, born Jan. 1, 1954, Evergreen Park, IL. Earned her associates degree in nursing from El Paso Community College, El Paso, TX in December 1995.

Assignments at St. Lawrence Dimondale Center, staff nurse; Lansing Community College, clinical instructor, Long Term Aide Program; substitute RN for Lansing Public Schools; staff nurse/occasional charge nurse, 6 Foster Rehab, Sparrow Hospital, Lansing, MI.

In 2003 she was awarded "Nurse of the Year," Rehab Services, Sparrow Hospital.

Married 28 years to Chuck Martin, they have four children: Charles Jr. of Chicago, IL; Adam of El Paso, TX; Steven currently serving active duty in the U.S. Army and stationed at Fort Rucker, AL; and Danielle is a junior at Catholic Central High School, Lansing, MI.

PAMELA MAULE, RN, CNOR, born Aug. 26, 1956 in Iron Mountain, MI. Throughout her 26 years of nursing she has worked in the operating room at Michael Reese Hospital in Chicago, IL, West Allis Memorial Hospital in Wisconsin, Baylor Medical Center in Dallas, TX and presently at Dickinson County Health-care System in Iron Mountain, MI.

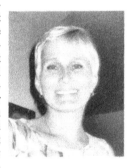

Personal awards: CNOR since 1990.

Other professional activities: Michigan Nurses Association, member and PAC Board, MNA staff council, member, Association of Operating Room Nurses, member and Superior Chapter secretary, Dickinson Area Catholic School Board, member and secretary.

Pamela is an active member of MNA local and state level, active in MNA staff council activities, and active in the Superior chapter of AORN. She enjoys attending state and national conventions as often as possible.

Education: Michael Reese School of Nursing, Chicago, IL, 1974-77; Classes at Northern Michigan University towards BSN.

Married to Douglas Maule of Kingsford, MI, they have three children: Patrick Mohundro, 18 years old and attending Kendall College of Art and Design, freshman year; Sean Mohundro - 16 years old and a junior at Iron Mountain High School; and Emily Maule, 8 years old and in third grade at Dickinson Area Catholic School.

Currently Pamela is an peri-operative nurse at Dickinson County Hospital and not only works in the OR but also the PACU and pre-op teaching. She enjoys working on monthly QA and call scheduling. Also enjoys being involved with her professional organizations and projects with her children. She is

a member of the Immaculate Conception Parish of Iron Mountain, MI and has recently become a lector during Sunday masses.

When in the fourth grade, her Uncle Duane, who is an orthopedic surgeon, married an operating room nurse. His stories about surgery always fascinated her. Since that time, she had always wanted to be an operating room nurse and still has that same enthusiasm for her profession.

MARILYN R. MCFARLAND, PhD, MSN, CTN, RN, born May 24, 1945. She is an adjunct faculty member at the Crystal M. Lange College of Nursing and Health Sciences, Saginaw Valley State University at University Center, MI, where she is currently serving as the coordinator of a special project, OPEN (Opportunities for Professional Education in Nursing), to recruit, engage and retain culturally diverse students in nursing.

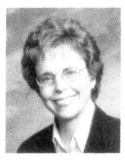

She received her PhD in nursing with a focus on transcultural nursing under Dr. Madeleine Leininger at Wayne State University in Detroit in 1995. Dr. McFarland, a transcultural nurse, has focused her professional work on the care and study of elders from diverse cultures in the U.S. and has presented her research findings about the culture care of elders worldwide. She is a former editor of the *Journal of Transcultural Nursing* and is an active member of the Transcultural Nursing Society, to which she has made many significant contributions. Dr. McFarland has also been a mentor to many students in the U.S. and abroad, making transcultural nursing meaningful and important in people care.

She has received many prestigious awards, including the Leininger Award presented by the Transcultural Nursing Society. She is an outstanding transcultural nursing researcher and educator who has helped to make transcultural nursing an exciting and relevant discipline.

Marilyn has been married 36 years to Dr. Rodney McFarland, an orthopedic surgeon.

SUSAN MELLA, born in Iron Mountain, MI, and is the mother of one daughter whom earned her BBA from St. Norbert College. She resides in her hometown of Norway, MI. Her nursing career started in 1976 right from high school. She attended Bay de Noc College and graduated in 1977 as a practical nurse.

Employment includes med-surg, ICU, OB, ER and geriatric nursing. To further her education she began taking classes at BDNCC towards her ADN, while working full time at Norway Hospital. In 1995 she graduated from BDNCC with her ADN. With this achievement she was hired to ICU at Dickinson Hospital.

She now works as a staff nurse in the Emergency Dept. In 2002 she was the recipient of a scholarship to attend the MNA convention, a wonderful experience. She now sits with Congress of Nursing Practice.

Certificates include BCLS, ACLS, PALS, TNCC. Her biggest inspiration to become a nurse lies with her family who stood by her all these years.

KRISTIN MELLON, RN, MSN, a native of northern Michigan, always wanted to be a nurse. She has a BSN from Michigan State University and an MSN from Wayne State University.

Membership and participation in the professional organization was cultivated by the faculty in her BSN program and she has been a participating member of the American Nurses Association since graduation.

Kristin had served as chapter president, secretary and delegate to the MNA, MNA involvement included the Medical-Surgical Practice Section, the Congress on Nursing Practice, the Board of Directors and delegate to the ANA. She was very honored to represent the MNA on the Governor's Commission on AIDS in 1982 and to be named Medical-Surgical Nurse of the Year.

After many years of practicing in acute care settings as a staff nurse, manager and clinical nurse specialist, she now focuses on ensuring appropriate care for our elderly in Long Term Care facilities.

MARTHA LEIGH MERKEL, born in Chelsea, MI, 1977; attended nursing meetings with her mother at age 3. In 1999, she received a BSN degree from the University of Pennsylvania.

While at school she was member of the nursing service group (Sub Rosa), a member of the softball team and a Hillman scholar. Critical care nursing sparked her interest and her senior clinical nursing was in a pediatric intensive care unit in New York City.

Family-centered care was the focus of her inquiry paper and continues to be an interest and a passion. She has worked as a home care case manager for Pediatric Services of America and is again practicing in the PCIU at C.S. Mott Children's Hospital at the University of Michigan. She is a member of Michigan Nurses Association. Currently she is pursuing an MS in Nursing Business and Health Systems at the University of Michigan. Nursing has provided her with opportunities for growth and leadership.

SANDRA MERKEL, born 1944 in Marcus, IA, received a BSN from the University of Iowa in 1966. She obtained her MS in psychiatric nursing from the University of Michigan in 1997. Pediatric nursing is her specialty and she is co-developer of a

behavioral pain assessment scale named the FLACC. She is a clinical nurse specialist on the pediatric pain services at C.S. Mott Children's Hospital.

In 2000, she received the hospital's first award for Excellence in Patient Care, Education and Research. She also received the "Nurse of the Year" award from Chapter 8 of the MNA in 2002. She has been active in MNA, serving in leadership roles at the chapter and state level. She enjoys planning creative continuing education programs and mentoring nurse leaders.

Traveling is an enjoyment and sailing with her husband was one of her most adventurous trips. Her daughter chose nursing as a career. She does not remember why she became a nurse, but she remains a nurse because of the challenges and rewards.

KRISTINE MICHAELSON, RN, Staff RN, born Dec. 17, 1952 in L'Anse, MI. Earned her AD at Michigan Tech. University. Employed as staff RN, Marquette General Health Systems, Orthopedics, ICU-Step Down Unit, Emergency Room, Recovery Room, Out-Patient Surgery. She has been at same hospital for 27 years.

Member MI Nurses, MNA, BOD (two years), E&GW Cabinet member (8 years) and recent member of congress. Received E&GW Award. She is president of Chapter 1; staff nurse Bargaining Unit, past chair; current grievance stewart and contract negotiator.

She has one son Kyle (age 11 years).

BARBRA MIKOWSKI, RNC, CNA, born April 25, 1942, Cadillac, MI. Earned her ADN from Northwestern Michigan College in Traverse City, MI; advanced study in rehab nursing at New York University, New York City, NY.

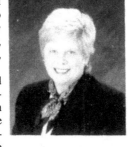

A licensed professional registered nurse in Michigan, she holds two certifications through the American Nurses Credentialing Center in Nursing Administration and as a Gerontological Nurse. She has worked with nurses in rural areas for 30 years in providing and coordinating workshops to enhance knowledge and skills regarding care of older adults. She serves on the Board of Directors for Michigan Center for Rural Health representing Michigan Nurses Association. She is member of the following advisory boards: Grand Traverse Pavilions - Long Term Care, Munson Home Health, Senior Volunteer Programs, Faith in Action Project and Great Lakes Community Mental Health Quality Improvement Council. Has been a member of MNA for some 30 years and served as chair

of the former Division of Gerontological Nursing. Was member of board of directors, including serving two terms as vice president. Currently employed by Catholic Human Services, Inc., Traverse City, MI. She manages multiple programs for older adults and their families in northwest Michigan, including Parish Nurses/Health Ministries.

Awards include Nurse of the Year for 1987 for Traverse City District Nurses Association; Recognition of Service in 1994 by MNA for serving on board of directors.

Her accomplishments include developing programs: Mental Health Services For Residents Of Nursing Homes and Long Term Care Facilities; Family Caregiver Support Services; Elder Abuse Awareness Programs and Dementia Caregiver Education.

Married in 1962 to James Mikowski, owner of JM Plumbing and Heating. They have two daughters: (1) Susan, nurse and health fitness, living in Laguna Beach, CA with husband Stuart Fraser and son Zane. (2) Elissa has degree in health fitness and lives in Traverse City, MI with husband Heath Holcomb, daughter Skylar and son Sterling.

DOROTHEA MILBRANDT, became an active member of the nursing profession in 1950, when she received her diploma from the Holy Family Hospital School of Nursing in Manitowoc, WI. Beginning as a staff nurse at Memorial Hospital in West Point, NE, she traveled to Ohio, Wisconsin, and finally to Michigan in 1968. Teaching and mentoring has always been a passion of Dorothea's — as associate professor at Michigan State University College of Nursing or during her 15 years as vice president for Nursing at Ingham Medical Center in Lansing.

Dorothea's list of appointments, honors, professional memberships, publications and presentations is lengthy. Her commitment to MNA and ANA, her professional associations, has been evident through the years — as a volunteer in many roles, including MNA President and Magnet Appraiser, and as an employee as the Associate Executive Director for Professional Association Services, and most recently Interim Executive Director.

Continuing education was also a constant in her career, with her adding a BSN and two master's degrees to her initial diploma education.

LARISSA E. MILLER, RN, born July 3, 1969, Mt. Clemens, MI. She is currently working as a nurse on the Cardiac Progressive Care Unit of Sparrow Hospital in Lansing, MI, where she has recently completed 10 years of service. She also serves as a BCLS instructor.

Larissa received both her bachelor's and master's degrees from Michigan State University and is a CNS in family practice.

She lives in East Lansing with her husband, David, a civil engineer, and their two sons, Nicolas and Daniel.

WILLIA M. MILLER, BSN, born in Olanta, SC, chose nursing as a career due to the lasting impression by a nurse relative during her early childhood. The observational experience at Harlem Health Center during her "training" at Harlem Hospital School of Nursing led her to choose public health as her field of interest. Willia joined the Detroit Dept. of Health in 1948, obtained a BSN in 1953, birthed a son in 1953 and was inducted into Sigma Theta Tau in 1954.

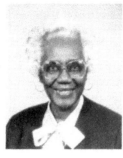

She joined Wayne County Health Dept. of Health in 1954, obtained the MPH at the University of Michigan in 1958 and attained the position of maternal and child health consultant before her retirement in 1981.

A lifetime member of MNA, Willia has served as chair person of the former public health section and secretary of the former maternal and child health section, as convention delegate and board member.

Willia's retirement years have been devoted to health related activities with a variety of community organizations including the American Cancer Society, American Red Cross, New Center Community Mental Health Center, Lula Belle Stewart Center for parenting teens, YWCA of Western Wayne County, Virginia Park Community Investment Associates, C.H. Wright Museum of African American History, American business Women's Association, Agencies of the United Methodist Church, among others.

She is a member of Chi Eta Phi Sorority and Alpha Kappa Alpha Sorority, having held local, regional and national offices and assignments in both. As a member of Second Grace United Methodist Church, she is a member of the choir and chairs the Missional Outreach Committee which conducts various health related ministries. Willia has received several citations for meritorious services and volunteerism from most of the listed agencies.

Willia, twice married, is now a widow and has two sons, seven grandchildren and one great-grandchild.

STEPHANIE MINERATH, earned her undergraduate nursing degree from the University of Wisconsin, Madison, where she began her professional career in inpatient pediatrics. Following a period of staff nursing, Stephanie earned her master's degree in pediatric nursing from Yale University in New Haven, CT.

Moving to Michigan in 1980, Stephanie worked as an instructor at the University of Michigan School of Nursing, and continued her clinical involvement by staffing at CS

Mott Children's Hospital at the U of M, which she did for many years. Most recently, she was in charge of the nursing orientation program at the University of Michigan for five years. Early on, Stephanie developed an ongoing interest in professional issues such as safe staffing, career development, and new nurse transition. Together with the Nurse Counselor at U of M, Stephanie developed a support program for new nurses including transition discussions, follow up meetings, NCLEX support, and mentorship. Stephanie is a certified rehabilitation registered nurse. She is an active member of the UMHS Nurse Retention Team.

Stephanie has a passion for the nursing profession, and recently created a quilt celebrating her first 25 years as a RN. The themes of the quilt reflect the themes of her career: children and families (who made the work so rewarding), teaching and learning (a lifelong habit), and people, including a multitude of friends and colleagues (who she both admires and appreciates).

Stephanie has been a frequent delegate to the Michigan Nurses Association Convention, and an active member of her staff council, The University of Michigan Professional Nurse Council. She is currently serving as UMPNC vice chair, and also works as an educational nurse specialist at UMHS.

LISA A. MITCHEM, RN, born June 26, 1953, Iron Mountain, MI. Earned her ADN at Bay de Noc Community College, Escanaba, MI and has med/surg. certification. She became a nurse because she has always been drawn to helping people. The nursing profession is a calling and her mother gave the encouragement she needed to pursue her dream of becoming a nurse.

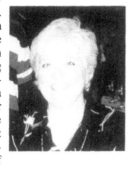

Employed as supervisor, Dialysis and Renal Clinic; staff nurse, Dialysis; week-end hospital supervisor at Dickinson County Health Care System. She received Employee of the Month in July 1996.

Active as DCHS Staff Council officer and MNA Congress Public Policy; Past MNA delegate, past ANA delegate and past UAN delegate.

Lisa and her husband John have three children: Andrew, Mary Kathryn and Adrian, and three grandchildren: Alex, Madelynn and Austin.

LINDA CAROL MONDOUX, born in Batesville, AR. Earned her BS in nursing at University of South Carolina in 1969; MS in medical-surgical nursing and Specialist in Aging Certificate, University of Michigan, 1981;

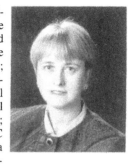

licensed in Michigan as a Nurse Practitioner and Nursing Home Administrator; ANCC Certification as a Medical Surgical Clinical Nurse Specialist; NADONA-LTC Certification as a Director of Nursing Administration in Long Term Care.

Linda served in the U.S. Navy Nurse Corps; was president of MNA from 1993-97 and over the years has served MNA in multiple capacities on the Board, Congress on Nursing and Healthcare Economics, Delegate to the ANA House, and various committees. She is Clinical Committee member for the RAND/UCLA ACOVE (Assessing Care of the Vulnerable Elderly) study and ANCC Magnet Program Appraiser.

Received Top Nurse of Michigan Award and Oakland University Finalist, Nightingale Award for Excellence in Nursing Administration in 1994, and MNA Outstanding Gerontological Nurse of the Year, 1990.

Other professional activities include founding and on-going member of the Michigan Chapter of the National Conference of Gerontological Nurse Practitioners and Michigan NADONA Board of Directors.

Her husband Bill is a financial controller at Ford Motor Co. Son, Dave, is a sophomore majoring in criminal justice at Michigan State University, and son, Tom, a US Naval Academy graduate and a U.S. Marine Corps lieutenant is currently in flight training.

Linda is president and sole proprietor of Strategies for Long Term Care in Farmington.

MARY KAY (WEALCH) MOORE, BSN, RN, MA, CDDN, MHA, was born near Ann Arbor, MI and has been interested in the healthcare field since the age of 6 when she began identifying with a nurse friend of her mother's.

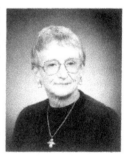

She was in the first class to graduate from the 4-year program at the University of Michigan School of Nursing in 1956 where she obtained her BSN. Her MHA came from Central Michigan University.

Since 1965, she has devoted her career to individuals with developmental disabilities and was involved in the establishment of the MNA Council for DD Nurses. She was presented with the 1986 ANA Excellence in Writing Award. She retired from Oakdale Regional Center, Lapeer, MI in 1989 and moved to

Georgia to become an independent consultant in the field of DD and currently works as an expert consultant/witness for advocate attorneys.

She was actively involved in the formation of the national organization, Developmental Disabilities Nurses Association, and was elected to a 3-year term as president, beginning Jan. 1, 2004.

Her husband died in 1986. She has two sons and five grandchildren, all of who live in Michigan. She is actively involved in church and community activities in the Peachtree City area.

BERNICE F. MORTON, Associate Professor Emeritus, born Aug. 29, 1923, Detroit, MI. Earned her MSN and BSN at Wayne State University, Detroit, MI, PhD Higher Education Administration Organization, University of Michigan, Ann Arbor, MI.

Assignments: Associate Professor Emeritus, Wayne State University; Director of Nursing, Comprehensive Health Services of Detroit; consultant of chronic diseases, Wayne County Health Dept., Detroit, MI; staff nurse, field teacher, Detroit Health Dept.; assistant director of nursing education, Metropolitan Hospital of Detroit; first visiting assoc. professor at the School of Nursing, Howard University, Washington, DC.

Awards include Mary Mahoney Award, American Nurses Association; Bertha L. Culp Award, Human Rights, Michigan Nurses Association, Minerva Educational and Development Foundation Inc., Founding Board of Directors, Project Healthy Living, Grant Coordinator and Project Dir.; Leadership Award in Community Health Nursing from MNA; Star Award from Detroit Black Nurses Association; Geraldine Doby Award for Nursing Excellence from DBNA; Michigan Black Nurses Mentorship Services Award; Spirit of Detroit Award and Pin; Distinguished Educator from Societas Docta, Inc.

Other activities include Sigma Theta Tau International Honor Society of Nursing, Inc.; Chi Eta Phi International Nurses Sorority and National Black Nurses Association.

Married and has two daughters and five grandchildren. She has given 50 years to the nursing profession and is currently working on *They Paved the Way,* a book about early black nurses.

ELIZABETH MARIE NELSON, born Sept. 2, 1922, Gladstone, MI. She went to Chicago, IL for nursing education at Augustana School of Nursing, 1941-44. Acquired nursing license from Illinois; also, applied and received from Michigan.

She worked at a hospital in Detroit for two years then went to work in U.P. Hospitals. She applied for New York license and worked there one and a half years, then returned to Gladstone and worked at local hospital, St. Francis.

Elizabeth was active in state membership

and active on local, state offices trying to get more memberships. Active local, state and US Nursing annual meetings as the local or state representative at meetings.

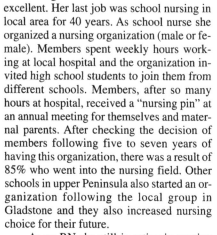

Experiences in nursing were excellent. Her last job was school nursing in local area for 40 years. As school nurse she organized a nursing organization (male or female). Members spent weekly hours working at local hospital and the organization invited high school students to join them from different schools. Members, after so many hours at hospital, received a "nursing pin" at an annual meeting for themselves and maternal parents. After checking the decision of members following five to seven years of having this organization, there was a result of 85% who went into the nursing field. Other schools in upper Peninsula also started an organization following the local group in Gladstone and they also increased nursing choice for their future.

As an RN she still is active in nursing activities, her church and Senior Center.

NANCY ROOK NELSON, born Sept. 14, 1928, Grand Rapids, MI. She attended Hope College, 1946-48, right out of high school. While at Hope, the Health Service Nurse presented a program to promote nursing as a profession. The Dean of the soon to be Wayne State University School of Nursing in Detroit spoke at this program presenting the advantages of "professional" nursing. She suggested that the best schools of nursing at that time were John's Hopkins University, Case Western Reserve and Yale University.

Nancy wrote to all three: Yale wrote back that she should contact them when she had her bachelor's; Case Western Reserve sent a 17 page application which she promptly filed in the wastebasket; John's Hopkins sent a one-page application and a one-page health form These she filled out and returned.

She was accepted to John's Hopkins. She then went to her grandfather who was paying her educational expenses and explained to him why she wanted to attend John's Hopkins, stating that it was rated as one of the best nursing schools in the Nation. He drew himself up to his full eighth grade education and said, "Don't you ever let anyone tell you that there is any better school than the University of Michigan." She did not know that the University had a nursing school but certainly found out in a hurry, applied and was accepted.

Memberships include ANA, MNA, Sigma Theta Tau, AWHONN, School of Nursing Alumni Association (life member and

served as officer), University of Michigan Alumni Association (life member, chairman of several committees and member of board of directors), Nursing History Society of the University of Michigan, University of Michigan School of Nursing Alumni Society, Member Medical Center Alumni Association.

Honors: Accolade, University of Michigan Alumni Association, 1979; Distinguished Alumni Service Award, University of Michigan Alumni Association, 1980; Centennial Recognition Award, University of Michigan School of Nursing, 1991; Proclamation, School of Nursing, 1994; Certificate of Recognition, University of Michigan School of Nursing Alumni Society, 1997.

She worked at the University of Michigan Health Systems for over 40 years in a variety of settings: 1952-94, University of Michigan as a staff nurse in various positions: Obstetrics/Gynecology, Neuropsychiatric Institute, Hypertension Clinic/Renal Clinic, University of Michigan School of Denistry, Research Nurse at School of Public Health Epidemiology Department and the Geriatric Arthritis Ambulatory Care Department.

TARA MICHELLE NICHOLS, BSN, ADN, BS, born Nov. 12, 1961, Detroit, MI. Earned her BS in psychology, Oakland University in 1987; ADN, Highland Park Community College, 1990; BSN, University of Michigan, 1994.

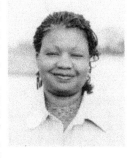

Assignments: Clinical Nurse II, Medical ICU, University of Michigan, 2002 to present; CNII Anesthesiology, Acute Pain Service, 1998-2001, U of M; CNI Home Med, 1997-98; CNI Cath Lab; CNI MICU, 1991-94.

Member of MNA, Chapter 8 board member; chairperson, Congress Nursing and Health Care Economics; chairperson, Nomination Committee; Program Committee Chapter 8, 2004-05 ANA delegate; 2002 – 2004 MNA delegate.

She was influenced by her grandmother, Carla Kirkland Harris, who was a midwife and birthed the majority of babies born in De Funiak Springs, FL, and also by her mother Lucy Lee Nichols. She always wanted to be a nurse, but every time she applied to nursing school she was pregnant and her admission was denied. Then at the age of 40, she attended Mary Grove College in Detroit, MI. While working two jobs and having nine children at home, she completed a nursing assistant program with straight A's and was top of her class.

Currently, Tara is working on Medical ICU at U of M, Pain/Sedation focus. She works part-time at Washtenaw Community College teaching fundamentals of nursing.

DANA ELANA NICHOLSON, RN, BSN, born May 27, 1964, Kalamazoo, MI. She earned her BSN at Nazareth College in 1986.

Assignments, all at Borgess Medical Center as float nurse, RN, 1986-87; ICU, staff RN, 1987-88; CSU, staff RN, 1988 to present; Critical Care Transport Nurse, RN, in 1990s.

Her greatest accomplishment was having her daughter, Samantha, after many years of trying which took many different procedures. She is now 13 months old.

GWENDOLYN SIMPSON NORMAN, PhD, RN, BSN, born April 17, 1953, Detroit, MI. She received her BSN from the University of Michigan in 1974, and having been awarded a full tuition scholarship to graduate school, received her master's of public health degree from U of M in 1976 at the age of 23. She then worked for three years as the nurse coordinator for the Parent Child Development Center, a research and demonstration project to help low-income mothers rear healthy, bright children.

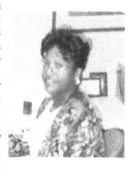

In 1979 she began as staff nurse in Labor and Delivery at Hutzel Hospital and in 1983 took the position of Perinatal Research Nurse Coordinator. Since 1991 she has been the research coordinator for the Maternal Fetal Medicine Unit network of the National Institute of Child Health and Human Development at Wayne State University.

In 2002 she received a Nightingale award in the category of Research and Education for the state of Michigan. She has been happily married for 27 years to Joe L. Norman, has two daughters, two adorable grandsons, and is currently completing her PhD in medical anthropology.

She credits her mother Lucille Simpson, RN, for being the perfect role model, and for her undying inspiration in the practice of her profession, and her father, Henry Simpson, for always making health a top priority.

DONNA NUSSDORFER, RNC, Certification in Maternal/Newborn Nursing, born July 12, 1946, Chicago, IL. Earned her diploma from Rush Presbyterian College of Nursing, Chicago, IL.

Assignments were in large and small hospitals, school nurse, hospice nurse and currently Public Health Nurse, Washtenaw County.

Donna has been married for 36 years and is the mother of four and grandmother of two.

SANDRA OLSON, Staff Nurse, RNC, ONC, born in Stambaugh, MI. She graduated

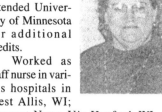

as valedictorian, St. Luke's School of Nursing, Duluth, MN and attended University of Minnesota for additional credits.

Worked as staff nurse in various hospitals in West Allis, WI; Newport News, VA; Hartford, WI; Crystal Falls, MI; Iron Mountain, MI, charge nurse for 10 years. Currently staff nurse, Radiation-Oncology at Dickinson County Health Care System, Iron Mountain, MI.

Received Excellence in Nursing Award, 1992 and 1995, Dickinson County Hospital. She is a member of ANA, MNA, ONS, Superior Chapter MNA. She has served on numerous nursing and hospital committees, attended fall and national conventions, ONS, Med-Surg Certification in 1994, ONS Certification in 2001 and ACLS Certification in 2003.

Sandra has been married 37 years and has two daughters.

MARIA ELIZABETH (BATEMAN) OSBORNE, born April 11, 1969, at Bronson Methodist Hospital in Kalamazoo, MI. Having a physician for a father, medicine and healthcare was a constant. Through grade school her compassion for others suffering developed into an interest towards nursing.

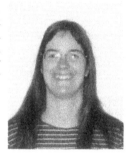

She went to Nazareth College in Kalamazoo, MI for a four year nursing degree. One memorable time in college was being able to tell her father she earned enough money from her nursing internship to pay for her senior year of nursing school without his assistance.

Maria "hospital-hopped" for five years after graduation, working adult medical-surgical, oncology, renal, pulmonary, neurology, orthopedics and pediatrics.

She found her "niche" in surgery at Lapeer Regional Hospital. Happily married and mother of three, she has practiced nursing for 12 years and worked surgical services for the last seven, caring for patients in all stages of surgery.

THERESA "TERRI" PREMO-PEAPHON, RNC (certified in inpatient obstetric nursing), Labor Organizer and Labor and Delivery Staff Nurse. She was born May 20, 1954, Saginaw, MI. Graduated from Mid-Michigan Community College with a practical nurse certificate; associate degree in

nursing from the University of the State of New York; bachelor's degree in union administration and leadership; graduated Cum Laude from the National Labor College. She is currently enrolled at the University of Baltimore, in legal and ethical studies masters degree program.

Terri, RNC, joined the MNA staff as a labor organizer in May 1999. Prior to coming to MNA Headquarters, Terri, a certified inpatient obstetrical nurse had been a staff nurse in labor and delivery at Sparrow Hospital in Lansing since 1989 and served as the staff council chairperson for seven years. She also served on the MNA Board of Directors, E&GW Cabinet and was chairperson in 1999. She has served as an ANA delegate since 1998 and played a key role in the development of the United American Nurses. She has served as a UAN delegate since 2000.

Terri received the E&GW Achievement Award in 1997. Other professional activities include chairperson of the Professional Employee Council of Sparrow Hospital (PECSH), MNA delegate, ANA delegate, UAN delegate and member of AWOHN.

Participated in the State Nurses Association Labor Coalition (SNALC), was involved in formation of the United American Nurses and worked for the AFL-CIO affiliation.

Married for 32 years, she has three daughters and four grandchildren. She is a lifelong member of the Catholic Church.

Terri has switched her primary focus to advocating for Nurses and Nursing. She assists RNs throughout the State to organize a union in their workplace. She also continues to work as a staff nurse in high risk obstetrics at Sparrow Hospital in Lansing.

KELLY PENROSE, RN, BSN, born Dec. 16, 1970, Ishpeming, MI. Received her BSN from Northern Michigan University. Employed at Marquette General Hospital since August 1992.

Every day she learns something new. After over 10 years of working as an RN, she still enjoys going to work every day. Patients are her priority.

Kelly and her husband Kurt have been married eight years and have a one-year-old son, Noah. Kelly works as a staff RN on a busy neuro/ortho unit.

JONELL M. PEPPIN, RN, BSN, born June 4, 1952, Robstown, TX. Earned her BSN at Incarnate Word University in 1974 and has continued to learn something new at work daily for 30 years.

Assignments include staff RN, Alice, TX; Newborn Nursery Supervisor, Austin, MN; staff RN,

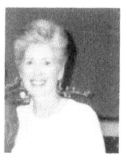

CCU, Ishpeming, MI; staff RN for 26 years, Marquette, MI, where she currently serves on four committees there.

Received Employee of the Month, MGH Hospital, 1990, 1995, 2000, MNA and E&GW Achievement Award in 2002.

Activities include Partners in Professional Nursing (10 years), Marquette General Hospital; Staff Council Negotiating Team; Retention and Recruitment Committee, MGH; RN Advancement Committee, MGH.

Accomplishments/Memorable Experiences: Texas NSA Chairman Scholarship Committee, 1973; TNSA State Scholarship recipient, 1972; attending her four children's college graduation; and pinning her daughter Tina during her nursing graduation ceremony.

Married 32 years to Paul Peppin, they have four children: Paul, Alan, Mark (wife Kristine) and twin daughters, Donna and Tina.

JANICE SUE STANTON-PETTENGILL, RN, BSN, MA, was born in Lansing, MI and followed in her nurse aunts' and cousins' footsteps and gradu-

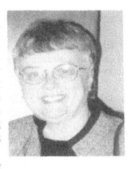

ated in 1964 from the University of Michigan. In 1983, she completed her master's degree at Michigan State University (MSU) and practiced nursing for 38 years.

Her nursing career began at Sparrow Hospital, where she quickly became the Medical Nursing Department Head. In 1978, she accepted a position with the new Clinical Center at MSU and soon became the Director of Nursing with additional responsibilities for the Olin Student Health Center. In 1987, she accepted a nursing consultant position with the Michigan Department of Public Health and continued as a nurse consultant in various state programs until retiring Nov. 1, 2002.

She has participated on numerous local, state, and national committees. Throughout her career, she was a leader and was instrumental in developing innovative programs to improve patient quality of care, service and life. In later years she focused on geriatrics.

She is a member of Sigma Theta Tau, MNA, and Michigan Society for Infection Control. In 2002, she received the MNA Excellence in Nursing Practice Award.

She is married and has a son and daughter-in-law.

LORI ANN POLFUS, RN, born July 29, 1962, Norway, MI. Attended Bay de Noc Community College for associate degree in nursing and emergency medical technician certification.

Assignments: staff nurse, relief charge nurse, DCHS; surgical floor then went to the

Ambulatory Care Unit cross-trained to home health; substitute school nurse, north central area schools; RN with a medical surgical certification, EMT.

Currently, she volunteers with Hermansville Rescue Squad and Ambulance Service, is CPR instructor and just recently started a new position in quality management.

Lori and her husband Ervin "Chip" have three children: Neil, Tyler and Seth.

SANDRA PONDER, ADN, RN, born 1966 in Detroit, MI. Attended Henry Ford Community College and got her ADN in 1989. She is still working on BSN.

She started working at Detroit Medical Center in 1988 while still in nursing school; worked three years at Medical ICU; one year surgical floor;

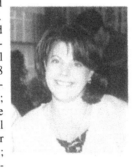

three years angiogram; three years community hospital; four years University of Michigan float staff, medical/surgical ICU and now neo-natal ICU.

Memorable experience was as a medical assistant student and a teacher wrote on her paper "You should think about going to nursing school." Her name was Cynthia Freeland Symington and Sandra will never forget her.

Sandra is married and has two stepchildren.

THERESA H. PORCH, born Jan. 7, 1958 in Michigan. Earned her BSN at Eastern Michigan University in 1987 and master's of art in healthcare administration in 2002. Accomplishment was completion of research paper (thesis), Occupation Stress as a predictor of job satisfaction.

Assignments: 1988 staff nurse SICU;

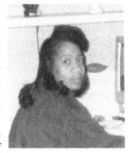

1989-2003, RN manager psychiatric nurse and presently working as quality improvement coordinator, Coordinate Women's Health Program.

Received the Landy Smith Achievement Award Christian Education. She is a member of the Healthy Mother, Healthy Baby Committee and member of NAFE.

Theresa and her husband Myron have a daughter, Ashley.

LORI POTTER, RN, born July 13, 1952. Earned her LPN in 1975 and RN in 1984 from

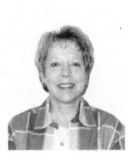

St. Clair County Community College. She has worked in nursing home, physician's office but most of the time has been hospital nursing and continuous position of neighborhood and family nurse.

Each day in nursing is a memorable experience and presents a new challenge. In the last 15 years she has "found her niche" in endoscopy, where she plans to remain for the remainder of her nursing career.

Lori and her husband Dennis have two grown children, Erin and Ryan, and one granddaughter, Anna.

KAREN POWERS, RN, BSN, born in Flint, MI. She earned her BSN from Northern Michigan University in 1977, and after graduation started her nursing career at Lapeer Regional Hospital.

Her first job was charge nurse on midnights in a med/surg ward. She stayed in that position until after the birth of her second child, then went part-time

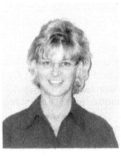

working as a float RN. She then took a recovery room job for four years and is now in radiology at Lapeer for three days a week.

Other activities include being on the negotiating team at Lapeer for the first contract and then again for this year's contract; filled in as vice president for one term for staff council; participated in a research project in the early 1980s; was a delegate to the MNA Convention several times; and BLS instructor for the Radiology Dept. at Lapeer.

Married to Patrick, a wonderful man, for 24 years, and they have two children, Jacob and Ashley. Karen is a member of Good Shepherd Lutheran Church, serves on the Fellowship Committee, chair member and member of Ladies Mission Society. She is also a booster for the Lapeer West Pom Pom team of which her daughter is a member.

JOAN PRENTICE, BSN, ADN, born June 20, 1956, Wayne County. Attended Saginaw Valley University for BSN and Delta College Saginaw for ADN. She received her Med/Surg Certificate in 1993.

Assignments: 1980-82, Bay Medical Center, GYN, Urology, Surgical; 1982-83, Saginaw General Hospital, Dialysis; 1983-86, Alpena General Hospital, Med/Surg.; 1986-95, Alpena General Hospital, nurse manager; 1995-2003, Alpena General Hospital

Surgical Pre-Admission; 2003-present, Alpena General Hospital, perioperative/infection control employee.

She won the Appreciation Award twice for serving on the Council of Nurse Managers, 1992 and 1996. Other activities include president, Staff Council, Alpena General, 1996-present and she is member of Michigan Nurses Association, 1983 to present.

Joan is the mother of three and grandmother of three (including a set of twins). Getting into nursing school was difficult for her. She was the second oldest of six children and the only girl. Both parents worked minimum wage jobs so she did qualify for the National Student Direct Loan. She remembers seeing in the paper that the Delta College was opening registration to the nursing program and her heart leaped with joy. She had wanted to be a nurse since she was in the sixth grade but never thought she would be able to due to money. The money was there and the desire, she just needed a school and waited in line from 2:00 a.m. to 2:00 p.m. She was #97 and they were only taking 100 applicants.

BETTE J. PROULX, RN, born April 17, 1957, Flint, MI. She earned her RN associate degree at St. Clair County Community College.

Bette worked 26 years at Lapeer Regional Hospital in Med/Surg, ICU and the last 18 years in OR.

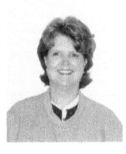

Married 25 years, she has a son Thomas (21) and daughter Erin (19). She enjoys activities with her family, golfing, scrapbooking, choir trips and recently started as a Mary Kay consultant.

GLORIA (BECKWITH) PUMMILL, RN, BSN, born June 9, 1931 in Detroit, MI. A 1949 graduate of Lowrey High School, Dearborn, MI. A 1953 graduate of St. Lawrence Mercy School of Nursing, Lansing, MI. She began at St. Lawrence Mercy Hospital. Upon returning home in 1954, she began her many years of work in the psychiatric field.

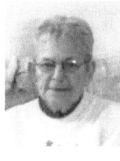

During her career she worked at the following facilities: St. Joseph's Retreat Psychiatric Hospital, 1954-55; Northville State Hospital, 1955-57; Wayne County

Psychiatric Hospital, 1959-66 and 1971-77; LaFayette Clinic, 1963; Dearborn Heights Convalescent Center, l966-71; Metropolitan Regional Psychiatric Hospital, 1977-80; Northville Regional Psychiatric Hospital, 1980-83; and Walter Reuther Psychiatric Hospital, 1983-97.

She received her BSN from Madonna College in 1976 while working full-time and caring for four children. Now retired, she enjoys spending time with her husband and family, especially her six grandchildren, and some travel. She has touched many with her compassion and love for people.

HELEN A. (LARSON) REHFELD, born Oct. 16, 1924, Shafer, MN. She entered Michael Reese Hospital School of Nursing Aug. 31, 1942, signed up for Cadet Nurse Corps when it was formed and was admitted into Corps July 1, 1943. She and her classmates were proud to have helped the war effort. She obtained her BSN from University of Wisconsin in 1958.

Assignments: Psychiatric, Michael Reese Hospital, Chicago; obstetrical-Sheboygan, WI, Memorial Hospital; assistant county nurse, Brown County, WI; county public health nurse, Mantowoc, WI; director, visiting nurse Association, Shebyoygan, WI; geriatric nurse, Frankenmuth Convalescent Center, Frankenmuth, MI; occupational nurse, General Motors, Saginaw Steering Gear, Saginaw, MI.

While working at Manitowoc she was a delegate to Ana Convention in Chicago – an impressive experience.

Married Frederick Rehfeld in 1959 – he passed away Aug. 1, 1999. She has a married daughter, Ruth Mesaros. Helen does volunteer work at church and school – Parents Teachers League, school library, school hot lunch, mobile meals, home delivered meals. She transferred her membership from WNA to MNA after she moved to Michigan.

EVELYN V. (REDWANZ) REINKE, Public Health Nursing Supervisor, born March 8, 1945, Saginaw, MI. She earned her diploma at Henry Ford Hospital School of Nursing; BSN, Wayne State University and MSN, Child Psych Nursing.

Assignments: Henry Ford Hospital, staff and head nurse; Beverly Enterprise, Staff

In-Service; Botsford General Hospital, staff nurse; Visiting Nurses Association of Detroit Community Health. She is currently public health nurse supervisor at Oakland County Health Division.

In 2003 she was awarded the Michigan

Public Health Association Leadership Excellence Award. Other activities include ANA delegate, MNA delegate, chair and vice chair Community Health Nurse Section, president of Oakland District Nurses Association, Sigma Theata Tau, Michigan Public Health Association and Governor's Task Force on childhood lead poison prevention.

Accomplishments include MPHA and APHA poster presentations, CDC lead conference speaker, co-ordinator of Oakland Childhood Lead Poisoning Prevention Program, Oakland County Immunization Action Program Co-ordinator; MNA Project Muscle Political Action.

She was married 37 years to Laverne Reinke, now deceased. They had two children, David and Leslie, and three grandchildren: Adam, Hailey and Brianna.

BETTY E. RICHARDS, RN, born Aug. 4, 1941, Cadillac, MI. She is a 1964 diploma program graduate of Hurley Hospital School of Nursing in Flint, MI.

Her first job as graduate nurse was at Sheldon Memorial Hospital, Albion, MI, caring for pediatric and post surgical clients in the 1960s; utilization review in the 1970s at Oaklawn Hospital, Marshall, MI; and currently working as staff nurse on the labor/delivery/post-partum/ nursery unit, Sturgis Hospital, Sturgis, MI.

In 2001 she was awarded the Faye Kerschner Nursing Excellence Award. Other activities include teaching pre-natal classes to expectant parents for many years at Sturgis Hospital. She loves being recognized on the street or in a restaurant by one of her OB clients and seeing how the baby has blessed this family.

VIRGINIA HILL RICE, PhD, RN, APN, BC, FAAN, Professor, Wayne State University College of Nursing and Karmanos Cancer Institute.

Ginnie was born in Webster, ME. Within three years of a Hartford Hospital School of Nursing Diploma, she earned a BSN at Boston University and taught and worked in Boston-area hospitals.

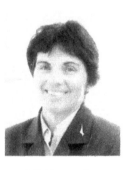

After moving to Michigan, she was awarded a MSN in Medical-Surgical Nursing from Wayne State and is a certified Clinical Nurse Specialist. She was elected to the Sigma Theta Tau. Ginnie completed both master's and doctoral degrees in social psychology at the University of Michigan.

Over the years she has had more than $5 million dollars in research funding, published numerous papers and books, and presented her work around the world. She has mentored some 60 master student projects, more than 30 doctoral dissertations, and three international students. Dr. Rice's research interests have been patient education, stress reduction, and behavioral change (e.g., tobacco use).

She serves on numerous professional and community boards, is married and has two sons.

NETTIE RIDDICK, LPN, ADN, MSN, was born in Selma, AL the fourth child of eight children. She decided early in life to become a nurse. Nursing school started in 1974 and continues today. Her nursing started with the LPN program. She entered and successfully graduated from Wayne County Community College with ADN in 1979, BSN from 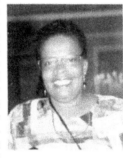 University of Detroit in 1991, and a MSN from the University of Phoenix in 1998.

She fell in love with neuroscience nursing during LPN clinical and has made it her career choice and is currently a nurse manager. She is certified in Medical/Surgical and Neuroscience nursing. She is a retired captain from the Army Reserves. She is currently president of Detroit Black Nurses Association, Inc., has professional membership in NBNA, Sigma Theta Tau, AANN, and ANA.

She was married, has one daughter, and three grandchildren. She is a member of New Greater Oregon, Mt. Moriah Baptist Church.

LINDA L. RIDLEY, RN, BSN, MA, born Aug. 17, 1948 in Cass City, MI. Earned her nursing diploma in 1969, Grace Hospital School of Nursing, Detroit, MI; BSN from Madonna College in 1977; and MA in health education and health science at Central Michigan University, Mt. Pleasant, MI.

Assignments: Grace Hospital, Detroit; 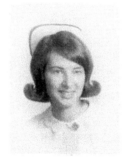 Botsford General Hospital, Farmington, MI; Northern Michigan Hospitals, Petoskey, MI as staff nurse; Central Michigan Community Hospital and Davis Clinic in Mt. Pleasant, MI as patient educational coordinator; Sparrow private duty nurse and Maxim Health Care, Lansing, MI. Currently she is doing home care and lecture series on "Living Beyond Disease," "Positive Spiritual Health for the Young and Old," "Not My God," and "You Have No Right to Abuse Women and/or Children."

Received Office Nurse Educator of the

Year Award in 1992 from American Association of Office Nurses; the Presidents Award from Great Lakes Society of Patient and Health Education in 1990; Outstanding Service Award from the American Heart Association of Michigan for the Mount Pleasant "Healthy Dining" in 1988.

Linda is Certified Health Education Specialist, 1990-98 and Certified Diabetes Educator, 1988-93.

BEVELY A. ROBERTS, MSA, BS, CRNA, RN, was born in Pine Bluff, AR to Thomas and Bennie Jean Brown. She is the oldest of six children. Bevely is the wife of Calvin and the mother of Calvin Jr. and Trina Nicole.

Bevely was first introduced to nursing as a future nurse volunteer at Flint Northern High School in 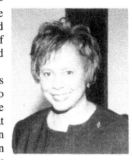 Flint, MI. She was awarded a scholarship to the Hurley Hospital School of Nursing in Flint by the Flint Urban League.

She graduated in 1968 from Hurley School of Nursing. In 1980 she received a BS degree from Mercy College of Detroit and at the same time fulfilled the requirements for graduation from the Mt. Carmel Mercy Hospital School of Anesthesia for Nurses. Since 1980 she has worked as a Certified Registered Nurse Anesthetists (CRNA). In May 2001 Bevely graduated with a MSA from Central Michigan University. She has earned a certificate in quality management and is also a licensed real estate salesperson.

Bevely is a member of Hartford Memorial Baptist Church, the American Association of Nurse Anesthetists, the Michigan Association of Nurse Anesthetists and the National Black Nurses Association. She has been a member of Chi Eta Phi Sorority Inc., Lambda Chi Chapter of Detroit, MI since 1987 and president of the local chapter from 2000 to 2003.

ELIZABETH "BETTE" O'CONNOR-ROGERS, LPN, ADN, BSN, born Aug. 16, 1958, Grand Rapids, MI. Earned her LPN in 1980 and ADN in 1985 at Grand Rapids Junior College; BSN from University of Michigan, graduating Magna Cum Laude in 1991.

She began her nursing career at Butterworth Hospital, Grand Rapids, MI on an ortho-neuro trauma floor for 12 years before coming to Visiting Nurses where she has enjoyed CHN for the last 12 years. She has worked as a case manager and, currently as an admission clinician in a variety of specialties such as rehab, hospice, general medsurg, infusion and wound ostomy. Currently

working Community Health Nursing for Visiting Nurse Services of Western Michigan as direct care staff in six counties in western Michigan.

Professional activities include chairperson of the VNSWM RN Staff Council, 1996-present; member of the E&GW Cabinet and the Impartial Committee of MNA; member Sigma Theta Tau International Nursing Society; has and continues to serve on multiple committees at each place of employment promoting improved day-to-day workplace life and standards of care.

Outside activities include serving as vice chairperson on both the Blythefield Acres Homeowners Association and the Blythefield Acres Pool, Inc. Boards; coordinator, Blythefield Acres Annual Splash-N-Dash 5k Run/Walk; coordinator of the Rose and Cornerstone Memorial Gardens and serves on the Building Committee for the addition of the Faith & Family Center at Assumption of the Blessed Virgin Mary Catholic Church (ABVM); coordinator of four annual Blood Drives for ABVM each year.

Bette was reared in a typical Irish-American household with eight siblings. She has been married 21 years to Scott with whom she has two wonderful children, Bridgett (10 years) and Connor (8 years).

In 8th grade, her Michigan history teacher gave them an assignment to report on a career. At that time he wisely advised them to try to choose their life career path as the career they reported on. Bette wanted to either be a nun or a nurse. Since she wanted to include children in her future she chose nursing and has never regretted it.

Her advice for a first year nursing student is to take a deep breath, relax, be patient and be ready to enjoy a life long journey of learning. Know it doesn't come clear right away but if you take it one step at a time, it will all fall into place and you will be hooked on the amazing science we call nursing.

KATHLEEN L. RONZEMA, RN, Staff Nurse, born Nov. 3, 1953, Borgess Medical Center, Kalamazoo, MI. Earned her ADN at Kalamazoo Valley Community College, CPR, BCLS instructor, ACLS.

Employed over 30 years at Borgess as an RN, 1997 to present, staff nurse, Endoscopy Lab and previously, 1975-97, Cardiac Rehab, Coronary Care Unit and Telemetry.

Memorable experience was being involved in the starting of the Coronary Intensive Care Unit at Borgess and all the wonderful nurses she has the privilege to know.

Awards include the Service Excellence Award. Other activities include CPR instructor, Borgess Medical Center, SGNA member and member of MNA since its inception at Borgess.

Married to Peter for 25 years and they

have two grown daughters and one daughter still at home and attending college.

AMY RORING, Clinical Nurse II, Staff RN, born Dec. 9, 1963, Chatham Ontario, Canada. Graduated with BSN, Madonna University in 1986.

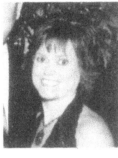

She worked in Yosuka Japan at a naval hospital and worked in San Diego at various hospitals. She has 18 years experience in medical telementry step down CCU experience. Currently she is working part-time, 24 hours, as staff RN on step down telementry at University of Michigan in Ann Arbor.

Married for 18 years, she has one son Joshua, 2-1/2 years old.

JANICE ROSENE, born in Battle Creek, MI and became a nurse after her aunt and uncle (both RNs) convinced her to take a Nurses Aide Course. They were right and she got her associates degree in nursing at Kellogg Community College.

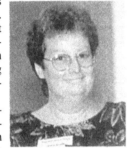

After relocating to Ishpeming, MI with her husband, she became a surgical floor nurse at Bell Memorial Hospital. Two children later, her family moved to Iron Mountain, MI where she worked ICU at Dickinson Memorial Hospital. During her early years at DCH a nurse, Elizabeth Willis, guided her through MNA staff council leadership roles. She became vice chair, chair, negotiation team member and chair of Professional Nurse Practice Committee. At the state level, she sat on MNA Restructuring Task Force and E&GW Cabinet.

She received the E&GW Cabinet Achievement Award in 2001. She is Superior Chapter secretary. She volunteers for the Knights of Columbus and St. Mary's Queen of Peace Church. She provides nursing care to patients in Cardiac Rehab.

MARILYN ROTHERT has been the Dean of the College of Nursing for the last nine years. The college enrolls approximately 800 students in the Bachelor of Sciences in Nursing (BSN), BSN-completion, Master's Science of Nursing, and PhD programs annually.

Dean Rothert received her Bachelor of Science in Nursing (BSN) from Ohio State University, her master's degree from Michigan State University in education psychology and her PhD from Michigan State University in education psychology.

Marilyn became a Fellow in the American Academy of Nursing in 1991. She continues to be a distinguished leader in nursing and has been recognized for her outstanding contributions to the nursing profession and to health care. Dean Rothert has been involved in research for over 20 years, including NIH funded research for women focusing on menopause and hormone replacement decision-making.

KATHY ROZEMA, BSN, RN, born March 13, 1978, Joliet, IL. Earned her BS in nursing, Western Michigan University in 2000 and is currently working on MS in community health at University of Michigan in Ann Arbor. After graduation she plans to practice as a family nurse practitioner in southwest Michigan.

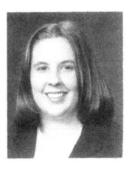

Worked as staff nurse in medical-surgical nursing at Borgess Medical Center, Kalamazoo, MI.

Awards include Lead, Link and Learn Scholar through the University of Michigan in 2003; numerous scholarships; graduated Sigma Theta Tau, 2003.

She served on MNA Congress on Nursing Practice, 2001-02 and MNA executive director, Search Committee, 2002-03. As a student she helped to advance the role of Michigan Nursing Student Association in the state and served the partnership with the Michigan Nurses Association.

She is married to Randy.

HELEN ROZNOWSKI, LPN, RN, BC, MSN, CDE, has a picture of herself at age four in a nurse's uniform, complete with cap. Frustration with physicians who didn't explain her son's childhood illnesses led to the desire to learn more about medicine. Helen became a LPN in 1978 and RN in 1985. She went on to complete her BSN and MSN.

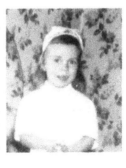

Helen currently works as a staff nurse in Endoscopy/Ambulatory Surgery/ PACU at Alpena General Hospital. She previously held positions of nurse manager and diabetes educator. While diabetes educator, Helen was honored by the American Association of Diabetes Educator with the prestigious "Nurse in Washington Internship" award. Helen received an "Outstanding Preceptor, 1992" award from student nurses at Alpena Community College. Helen has been a part-time instructor at ACC. She holds the office of MNA Staff Council Chairperson, and is the Chapter 2 Treasurer and representative to the MNA Board.

REBECCA SATOVSKY RUBIN, RN, BSN, born Aug. 30, 1981, Detroit, MI. She always knew that she wanted to attend the University of Michigan in Ann Arbor. When she was filling out her application her parents (mom in particular) suggested and pushed the idea of applying through the Nursing School. She was apprehensive but after several nursing classes her interest remained.

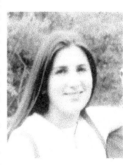

Four years later she developed enthusiasm and respect for the profession and proudly became a RN with a BS in nursing.

She attended University of Michigan, School of Nursing in Ann Arbor, graduating Cum Laude; also received Dean's list and university honors for multiple semesters.

Nursing school provided many challenges, but she succeeded because of teachers who believed in her, fellow students who kept her going and amazing family and friends that always supported her.

Her boyfriend, Michael Schostak, is a first year medical student at Wayne Medical School and hopes to graduate with a MD and MBA. He has respect for nursing and together they learned a lot from each other. Currently, Rebecca is participating in the Beumont MEO/SWG RN internship in neurology and is looking forward to a rewarding career in nursing and taking advantage of the many things it has to offer.

JUDITH POLACHEK SADLER grew up on a farm in Engadine, MI and planned on becoming a nurse from the time she can remember. She joined the first class of nursing students at Northern Michigan University graduating in the summer of 1971. Judy began her career in nursing with an internship at the Medical College of Virginia in Richmond, moving to the VA system in Richmond and Ann Arbor before completing her master's degree in nursing administration from the University of Michigan in 1978. Judy worked for several years in administrative positions in Michigan, South Carolina and Wisconsin before returning to bedside nursing while completing her PhD at the University of Wisconsin in Milwaukee in 1995. Judy has spent the last 13 years in higher education as a faculty member in schools of nursing. She currently is an assistant professor of nursing at the school of nursing at Western Michigan University.

NANCY C. SAYNER, DNSc, RN, born June 3, 1935, Cleveland, OH. Earned her BSN at University of Michigan and MS and DNSc at University of California in San Francisco.

Assignments include associate dean, Texas Christian University; senior year faculty coordinator, Duke University; senior year faculty, University of California; 14 years of various clinical roles.

Awards include Outstanding Faculty Member, UCSF in 1972 and Emeritus Faculty, Texas Christian University. She served 21 years (active and reserve) in the US Navy Nurse Corps, and received the Navy National Defense and 20 year medals.

Nancy is currently semi-retired and co-owner of Woodcraft Gift Shop.

MARY KAPENGA-SCHEERHORN, BSN, MSN, RN, always wanted to be a nurse. After 30 years as a RN, she reflects upon her professional career with great satisfaction. In 1972, she graduated from Bronson Methodist Hospital School of Nursing with her diploma degree.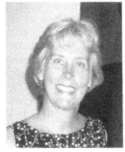

In 1986, she achieved her BSN from Grand Valley State University and in 1993, her MSN from Andrews University.

Currently, she shares her passion for nursing as an assistant professor of nursing at Hope College. She is a sexual assault nurse examiner for The Center for Women in Transition in Holland and works prn in the Emergency Department at Holland Community Hospital.

Previous nursing roles she held includes Director of Emergency Services, Nurse Educator, Trauma Nurse Coordinator, Clinical Supervisor of Emergency Services, ENPC instructor, and staff RN in the Emergency Department, Critical Care and Medical/Surgical Units.

The following are just a couple of highlights in her nursing career. As the Trauma Nurse Coordinator for Holland Community Hospital, 1997, she was recognized for her active involvement in the accreditation as the first Level III Trauma Care Facility in the state of Michigan.

In 1998, she was awarded two grants ($15,000 and $22,000) for implementation of the Lakeshore SAFE KIDS Coalition.

In 1998, she was the project coordinator for the Ambulatory Addition of a new Emergency Department and urgent care center at

Holland Community Hospital, which was part of a $23.5 million building project.

As a contributing member of the MNA, she served four years as the treasurer and three years as a delegate for the Lakeshore Chapter, She is the Hope College Department of Nursing faculty counselor for Sigma Theta Tau International, Kappa Epsilon Chapter. She serves on Board of Directors for Hospice of Holland and chairs their Ethics subcommittee.

Mary lives in Holland and is married to Mark and has two beautiful boys, Curtis (age 23) and Steven (age 17).

LAURA A. SCHMIDT, MSN, RN, born in Philadelphia, PA. Earned her ADN in 1976 and BSN in 1983 at Gwynedd Mercy College in Gwynedd Valley, PA; and MSN in 1997 at Northern Michigan University in Marquette, MI.

Assignments: staff nurse in orthopedics, neourosurgery, pediatrics and ER; staff development instructor; manger of medical/surgical unit; director of Acute Care Services; began teaching in 1994 at Northwestern Michigan College in Traverse City and director, Nursing Programs & Allied Health.

Awards: NMC Foundation Excellence Award and Outstanding Regional Leadership Award.

Other: past president of Michigan Council of Nursing Education Administrators (MCNEA); member MONE, Sigma Theta Tau and Phi Kappa Phi.

She enjoyed working as a leader with the Boy and Girl Scout organizations with her children, and mission work with the high school youth at her church each summer.

Married 26 years and has a son who is a senior at Central Michigan University and a daughter who is a high school senior.

Currently she is a member of Sacred Heart Catholic Church; Vice Chair, Pastoral Council; High School Youth Minister; and completing a post masters certificate from Grand Valley State University for a Family Nurse Practitioner Certificate.

KERRI D. SCHUILING, PhD, WHCNP, CNM, is the associate dean for nursing at Northern Michigan University's School of Nursing. She became the head of the nursing department in 1999. Kerri has a baccalaureate degree in nursing (Northern Michigan University); a master's in advanced maternity nursing (Wayne State University) and a PhD in nursing (University of Michigan). Additionally she is a certified nurse midwife (Frontier School of Midwifery and Family Nursing) and women's health nurse practitioner. Kerri has over 25 years of practice and education experience. She has authored several articles and presents internationally on her research, which looks at providing comfort to laboring women. Presently she is co-authoring a textbook on women's gynecologic health.

PATRICIA S. BERGER-SHILEY, BSN, Staff Nurse, born Aug. 8, 1950, Owosso, MI. For as long as she can remember she wanted to be a nurse. Her grandma and a great-aunt were nurses. She earned her BSN at Nazareth College, Kalamazoo, MI.

Assignments as staff nurse, supervisor, labor representative for MNA from 1989-97 and home care. Currently she is staff nurse in long term care.

In 1887 she received the E&GW Award. She is also active in district, state and national Association and has attended many state and national conventions. She served as president of Michigan Student Nurses Association, 1971-72. She took care of a man at home with muscular dystrophy on a ventilator, who taught her so much about life.

Patricia is married and has three children.

CHRISTINA SIELOFF, BSN, MSN, CNA BC, born in Detroit, MI, became interested in becoming a registered nurse, as a young girl, when reading fiction with nurses as leading characters. She attended Wayne State University for her BSN and MSN (major: nursing administration and minor, psychiatric and mental health nursing with children and adolescents); and PhD in nursing (focus: nursing group power). She is certified as a nurse administrator (CNA BC) through the ANCC.

Her clinical specialty is psychiatric nursing. She has worked primarily in inpatient settings, with patients across the lifespan. She became interested in teaching in 1992, while working with a community agency. Since 1993, she has worked at Oakland University's School of Nursing and currently an associate professor.

She has been active in the Southwest (formerly Detroit) Chapter, State and National levels of MNA and ANA for over 20 years. She is married to Ron Leibold, a teacher of second through fifth grades, who focuses on improving children's reading.

LUCILLE SIMPSON, RN, born March 2, 1931, Gay, GA. When she was a 16-year-old farm girl in Georgia, Lucille had her brothers held an injured pig, while she sewed it up. From that point on, everyone knew she'd be a nurse.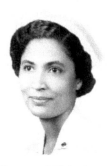

After marriage, a move to Detroit, and the birth of two daughters, she attended Detroit Practical Nursing Center. She earned the second highest score in the state. She began as a LPN in obstetrics in 1959 at Detroit Memorial Hospital, and moved to Herman Keifer Hospital in 1961, working with tuberculosis patients.

At Detroit Receiving Hospital in 1962, she assisted in opening the first hemodialysis unit in the state. She worked there until the unit closed, loving the job, the challenges and her patients. She returned to school at WCCC, earning her associates degree in nursing. When she took her state boards in 1982 to become an RN, she scored in the top 5%.

Her official retirement in 1994 did not end the skillful and compassionate practice of her profession. After having breast cancer in 1993 she began working weekly as a volunteer in a Karmanos Community outreach center, and with their speaker's bureau. She freely shares her time and nursing skills with family members and friends who are ill, and gives relief and support to their families. Because of her selfless acts of love, she was presented the Smooth Jazz V98.7 Acts of Kindness Award in 2002. To many, many people, she is an angel on earth.

DEBORAH A. SLEIK, Kingsford, MI, holds a master of science degree in nursing from northern Michigan University, Marquette. She was named the 2003 "Outstanding Graduating Graduate Student" for nursing. Her practicum work dealt with critical thinking skills and preferred learning styles of first year nursing students.

She currently works at Dickinson County Healthcare System in Iron Mountain as an OB nurse, prepared childbirth education instructor, and a hospital-based Neonatal Resuscitation Program instructor. She also teaches classroom, clinic, and lab classes in the nursing program at Bay de Noc Community College, Escanaba.

She serves on the Dickinson-Iron Intermediate Schools Advisory Board for Health Occupations and the Fiscal and Physical CI team at Bay College. She is a member of Our Savior's Lutheran Church, Iron Mountain. She was married to Dennis who passed away from cancer in February 2003. She has three adult children: Brad and his wife Colleen, Brian, and Dan.

MARILYN SMIDT, BSN, MSN, born in Fremont, MI. She earned her BSN at MSU and MSN at WSU. She is Director of Nursing Programs, Grand Rapids Community College.

Other activity includes Sigma Theta Tau, MNA, MCNEA, NLNAC, Commissioner and Program Evaluator.

Marilyn is married to Corwin E. Smidt and they have children, Andrea and Cory.

CAROL A. SMITH, Member Records Representative, born July 31, 1952 in Lansing, MI. A staff member for 29 years, Carol began her career with the MNA as a secretary in the Economic and General Welfare Department and filled that role for 14 years. Her current responsibilities include answering membership-related questions and solving problems for members, especially those in the

smaller bargaining units. She also invoices and posts dues payments, helps create reports, maintains the currency of records pertaining to bargaining units, and fulfills requests for mailing-list labels.

Prior to joining the MNA staff, Carol worked as a secretary for a paper company. She has attended classes at Lansing Community College.

SANDRA K. SMITH, RN, BSN, MSN HNC, CHTP, born in Highland Park, MI became interested in nursing at age 5 when she visited the hospital and watched the nurses care for her grandfather. She received her RN from Mott Community College, her BSN from the University of Michigan-Flint (UMF) and her MSN from Saginaw Valley State University. She worked in hospital nursing for 15 years and currently teaches nursing clinicals at the UMF. She is a faculty advisor to the Student Nurse Association at UMF and received the "Faculty Advisor of the Year" award from the Michigan Student Nurse Association in 2000.

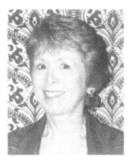

She is currently president Of Chapter 4 of the MNA, past-president of the GLS District, and has served in other board positions at the local and state level. She received the GLS District "Nurse of the Year" award in 1997. She values the rewards of her active involvement with her professional organization.

She is a Certified Holistic Nurse, Certified Healing Touch practitioner and owner of Complementary Care, LLC. Currently she is conducting research in the use of guided imagery for pain and anxiety management at a local medical center. She believes and enjoys the fruits of family connections, tennis, yoga, exercise programs, gardening and reading that nourish her body/mind/spirit.

NANCY HODGE-SNYDER, RN, Operating Room Supervisor, born March 19, 1922, Safford, AL. Graduated Clark High School and Columbus Medical Center School of Nursing, Columbus, GA.

She came to Kalamazoo, MI, in 1944, applied and was accepted at Bronson Methodist Hospital. She worked in the operating room on all three shifts and eventually became supervisor on the afternoon shift. After 14-1/2 years at Bronson, she worked at Borgess Medical

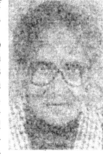

Center for nine years. She then went into private duty work for 10 years before retiring.

Awards include Certificate for Assistant with Brite Lite Choir, Certificate of Appreciation from Second Baptist, and Certificate of Leadership as a founding member of Columbus Medical Center Nursing Alumni.

Other activities include being volunteer nurse for Planned Parenthood of Kalamazoo, volunteer nurse for Boy Scouts of America Camp (through the Police Dept. of Kalamazoo), and church nurse at Second Missionary Baptist Church.

Memorable experience was being the first black RN at Bronson Methodist Hospital and being a founding member of the Columbus Medical Center School of Nursing Alumni.

Nancy is a widow and has two sons, Vincent and Larry Hodge; daughter Carolyn Hodge; and two granddaughters, Sasha and Zita Hodge-Wren. Retired, she is currently secretary of Columbus Medical Center Nursing Alumni.

REMEDIOS ALVAREZ SOLARTE, MSN, RN, NP, born and educated in the Philippines and migrated to the United States in 1972. She has been teaching medical surgical nursing at Oakland Community College for the past 24 years.

She obtained her diploma in nursing from Far Eastern University, Manila, Philippines in 1962 and consequently her BSN. She completed her MSN at Wayne State University, Detroit, MI in 1982. She was a member of the Michigan Board of Nursing. She is the 2003 Nightingale Awardee for Education/Research sponsored by Oakland University.

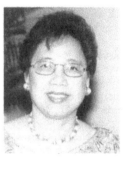

She is founding member and past president of the Philippine Nurses Association of America, the national organization of Philippine nurses in the United States. She sits in the Advisory Council of both the national organization and the Philippine Nurses Association of Michigan of which she was past president.

She is married and the mother of two adult children. She has two grandchildren, ages six and three.

PATRICIA C. STANAK, RN, born Oct. 1, 1926 in Wyandotte, MI. Assignments were at St. Joe's ER, Nursery and Pediatrics, 1947-55; Wyandotte's General Hospital ER, 1955-60; Oral Surgeon's Office, 1960-64; Ford Motor Co., 1964-89. She retired from Ford as senior nurse at Livonia Transmission Plant.

Awards include CPR Commendation,

Fire Safety Commendation and graduated with highest honors, Dale Carnegie Course.

She took several CEU courses during her 42 years in nursing and had a very satisfying and fulfilling career. Patricia has attended National AAOHN conventions at Disneyland, Atlanta and Los Angeles.

Single (never married), she shares a home with her brother and sister. Their parents are deceased.

JENNIFER JOHNSON STEINER, ADN, BSN, Clinical Nurse, born Feb. 24, 1956, Traverse City, MI. She earned her ADN at Northwestern Michigan College in 1977 and BSN in 1980 at University of Michigan.

Assignments include GN/RN June-October 1977, Monson Medical Center, RN (ADN and BSN) University of Michigan Medical Center 4E Mott, Adult Leukemia, 1977-78; 7W Mott, pediatric infectious diseases, 1978-81; pediatric hematology/ONC outpatient and infusion services, 1981-present. She currently works part-time in Pediatric Infusion Services, Myclodysplasia and HIV clinics at University of Michigan Medical Center.

Married and has three children, ages 18, 16 and 13. Her husband is employed by U of M.

KAREN KAISER STEPANIAK, Staff Nurse, RN, born Sept. 28, 1948, Alpena, MI. Influenced by her dad to become an RN, she received her diploma from St. Joseph Mercy Hospital, Flint, MI, in 1970.

Assignments include staff nurse/charge nurse, Neonatal Intensive Care Unit, St. Joseph Mercy Hospital, Ann Arbor, MI; staff nurse/charge nurse, Alpena General Hospital, Alpena, MI.

Other activities include MNA and ANA. Married, no children, she is now retired and winters in Apache Junction, AZ.

GERTRUDE L. PLOUG-STAPISH, born July 19, 1911, Bay City, MI. In June 1930 she graduated from St. Michaels HC, Flint with a Latin Scientific Diploma and in September 1930 entered Mercy Hospital School of Nursing, graduating in May 1933. Also took three year course study for diploma and courses at Delta College and SUSU.

She did private duty nursing, 1933-48 and much volunteering in air raid drills and health clinics. She participated in Women's Health Study; was active in Bay District Nurses Association, now Bay Central Chapter 8 MNA; and was delegate to state conventions. In 1948 she returned to hospital staff nursing and retired in 1976 from Bay Regional Medical Center.

In November 1933 she married Edward Stapish who passed away in 1971. Daughter Joyce is a piano teacher; Patt is a secretary; son Ed Jr. is retired from State Farm Insurance; and daughter Molly Jo, CNS RN,

teaches part-time at College of Nursing, MSU and works at Sparrow Hospital.

LINDA KAY (TANNER) STRODTMAN, born March 24, 1944 in Reno, NV, graduated from Hurley Hospital School of Nursing in 1965, Michigan State University in 1967, The University of Michigan in 1970 and Wayne State University in 1994, PhD. She is one of the first three clinical nurse specialists at University Hospital (1970) and is an

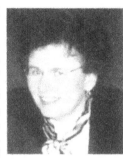

assistant professor at the UM School of Nursing. Her present clinical practice focus is palliative care.

She is married to Scott Strodtman and mother to Andrew and Susan.

Linda, co-founder, president and archivist of the Nursing History Society of The University of Michigan, has received many awards including: Excellence in Nursing, Sigma Theta Tau, (1982, 1999), UM School of Nursing Centennial Recognition (1991), American Nurses Foundation Scholar, 1992-1993, National Endowment for the Humanities for study on the history of death in America at Columbia University (1998), Mae Edna Doyle Teacher of the Year (1999), and the first Hurley Hospital School of Nursing Distinguished Alumni, 2002.

Linda collects nursing ephemera and antique and modern nurse dolls.

PHILIP SWEET, Assistant Nurse Manager, Clinical Coordinator, Nurse Manager, born Jan. 14, 1950 in Detroit, MI. He got his BA in psychology at Oakland University in 1972; diploma at Harper School of Nursing, 1974; and MSN, Wayne State University in 1982.

Assignments as staff nurse, Med/Surg, ER, Psych at Harper Hospital, 1974-87; instructor at four schools of nursing, 1975-96

Awards include Outstanding Young Man of America and Sigma Theta Tau since 1984. Currently he is MNA secretary/treasurer of Bargaining Unit at Alpena General Hospital. Active in 12 step recovery groups. Working with patients and students and seeing people recover is very rewarding.

He lives with his wife Maureen on Lake Huron and they have thee daughters: Jennifer, Aimee and Emile, and three grandsons: Christopher, Kaden and Ethan. Philip is currently working as nurse practitioner of Behavioral Health Service, Alpena General Hospital in Alpena, MI.

LISA SYLVEST, born in Detroit, MI and became interested in health care when she was in high school. She attended Michigan

State University and received her BSN in June 1980.

Lisa has been a member of MNA since 1980. She has been a member of Bylaws Committee, and under the old structure, the

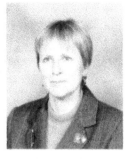

Med-Surg Practice Council. She has served as a Chapter 8 Delegate to MNA and as a MNA delegate to ANA and UAN.

At the staff council level, she has served as UMPNC secretary and representative. Lisa has worked at the University of Michigan Health System since 1981, currently practicing in Outpatient gastroenterology. She lives in Dexter, MI with her two children.

LINDA TAFT, LPN, RN, born in Grosse Pointe, MI and became interested in helping others after being hospitalized at age 12. Remembering the care and compassion of the nurses who cared for her, she embarked upon an adventure in health care that evolved from Candy Striper to Nurse's Aide to LPN and continues as an RN today.

She graduated from Shapero School of Practical Nursing (1976) and then attended St. Clair County Community College to obtain an associate's degree in Nursing (1993).

She was honored with SCCCC's "Certificate of Recognition" (1993), was a nominee for Oakland University's Nightingale Awards for Nursing-Staff Practice (2003) among many other honors in her career.

She has served as delegate, secretary and president for the Southeast Chapter of MNA.

Linda and her husband, Curt, live in Clinton Township with daughter Julie. She works in Surgical Services at North Shores Hospital, Harrison Township.

NUTRENA WATTS-TATE, MS, RN, CPNP, born July 7, 1974, Detroit, MI. She earned her BSN at University of Michigan in 1996; MS at University of Michigan in 2000; and is currently enrolled at Wayne State University in PhD Program.

Assignments as pediatric nurse practitioner, Sickle Cell Center, Children's Hospital of Michigan.

Awards include Ellen H. Topurek Excellence in Pediatric Nursing in 1996. Other activities are Sigma Theta Tau, National Black Nurses Association, National Association of Nurse Practitioners, MNA, IASC PAN International Association of Scale Cell Program Assistants and Nurses.

Her accomplishment was finishing the Walt Disney World Marathon Jan. 11, 2004. Nutrena and James have been married one and a half years.

AGNES HENIGE-TAYLOR, MSN, BS, born Oct. 30, 1942, Flushing, MI, and encouraged to become a nurse by her grandmother.

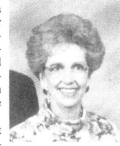

She's a 1963 Hurley Diploma graduate, got her BS degree at Central Michigan University in 1966 and MSN in parent-child nursing in 1986 at Wayne State University.

Agnes taught nursing (all subjects) for 25 years, 1966-90; did camp nursing in summers for Girl Scouts; school nursing for special needs children; was assistant director of Hurley School, 1990-95.

Awarded GLS District Nurse of the Year Award in 1996, Employee of the Month at Hurley Medical Center in December 1995. Other activities include MNA member approximately 35 years, Holistic Health Care Focus, chaired Legislative Committee of GLS District and was also treasurer and a convention delegate for GLS. She was facilitator of Grief and Loss Group (Beginning Experience) for 10 years and member of Big Little Sisters of Genesee County for 10 years.

Married, husband retired school teacher. Agnes is member of St. Roberts Catholic Church and is a Eucharistic minister and serves on other committees also. She is currently working part time with special needs children, traveling, and enjoying her two grandchildren.

PEGGY TAYLOR, born in Jackson, MI wanted to be a nurse since she was eight years old. She graduated from University of Michigan School of Nursing in 1981. One month after graduation, Peggy moved to South Carolina and began working at Conway Hospital. After passing nursing boards, she was placed in charge of a Med-Surg floor. One of the biggest challenges was learning to start IV's and draw blood on patients with difficult to locate veins.

Peggy worked at Children's Hospital in Texas for a year, then moved back to Michigan and worked the NICU at University of Michigan Hospital for one and a half years. Peggy has worked at the Jackson County Health Department (JCHD) as a Public Health Nurse for 18 years. She works in the Children's Special Health Care Services program.

Peggy is the Vice President for the JCHD's Nursing Association Prior to that she was the secretary-treasurer for 15 years. Peggy is married and has two children.

SHERRY JO THELEN, RN, Staff Nurse, born June 21, 1953, Ionia, MI. Earned her associate degree at Ferris State University in 1973. Assigned as staff nurse at Blodgett Memorial Hospital, 1973-79, Shorehaven Nursing Home, 1981-82.

Sherry is MNA grievance representative at NOCH. She and her husband William have two sons, Jeremy and Matthew. Currently, she is staff nurse in PACU at NOCH, Grand Haven, MI, 1982 to present.

JOYCE M. FERRIER-THEWALT, RN, CNOR, BSPA, born Sept. 10, 1941, Clifford, MI. Graduated North Branch High School, North Branch, MI; Evangelical School of Nursing, Detroit, MI, Diploma Program; St. Joseph Mercy College, Portland, ME, BSPA degree (hospital administration).

Assignments 1962-68, staff nurse OR, head nurse then supervisor OR, Deaconess Hospital; 1978-99, Mercy Hospital aka Samaritan Hospital; 2000-01, staff nurse Out-Patient Surgery Center, Siani Grace Hospital; 2001-present, Lapeer Regional Hospital as staff nurse, surgery.

She obtained CNOR in 1979 and attended Congress at OR Nurses Convention several times as a delegate. Also active in Lake Shore Chapter (Detroit area) and acted as secretary, vice president, president for chapter, and assisted in planning seminars for the chapter.

Her parents are Loyd and Sylvia Ferrier and she has a brother (married with three children). Joyce and Arnold have been married 32 years. He is a real estate referral specialist.

LIZABETH THOMAS, Clinical RN, born May 30, 1955 in Kalamazoo, MI. Earned her ADN at Kirtland Community College in 1986. She worked Med/Surg for four years, dialysis for 11 years and cardiology for three years.

Lizabeth was certified nephrology nurse and current ACLS. She loves nursing – it has been a very satisfying career to her. Currently she is working in noninvasive cardiology, Sparrow Hospital, Lansing, MI.

She is married to Jim and they have daughters, Jennifer and Cheryl, and granddaughters: Samantha, Alexandria, Gwendolyn and Taylor.

PATRICIA THORNBURG, RN, born Oct. 8, 1947, Detroit, MI. Earned her BSN at University of Michigan; MS, Ohio State University; and PhD (nursing), University of Cincinnati. She is a member of MNA Chapter 8, MNRS, and Sigma Theta Tau. Currently, she is on Wayne State University faculty.

PATRICIA W. UNDERWOOD, PhD, RN President of MNA, 1989-93, during her presidency, members promoted the view of

MNA as a single purpose organization that would advance the profession using multiple effective strategies. New bargaining units were organized, a new headquarters was built in Okemos, MI; Medicaid guidelines

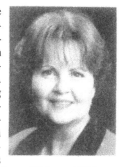

were written to reimburse FNPs and PNPs as independent practitioners, the Health Professionals Recovery Act was passed, and the Coalition of Michigan Organization of Nurses was formed to pursue a common political agenda. Dr. Underwood was COMON's first president.

She received her BSN at Duke University, an MS in Maternal-Child Nursing from Boston University, and a PhD in Nursing Research from University of Michigan. Her first love was staff nursing in pediatrics and obstetrics and further education was used to leverage the power of the staff nurse in achieving supportive work environments and quality care. She co-founded the Kalamazoo Nursing Research Collective to help staff nurses use research to their advantage.

An educator, researcher, and health policy expert, Dr. Underwood's leadership positions include president of Chapter 5 DNA and secretary and first vice president of the American Nurses Association. Her contributions to nursing have been recognized through the MNA Search for Excellence award and awards from Duke University, the Midwest Nursing Research Society, Kappa Epsilon Chapter of Sigma Theta Tau, and the American Journal of Nursing.

ELEANOR (TROMP) VERLEE, BS, MA, TC, born Aug. 12, 1927. Attended Mercy Central, Grand Rapids, MI for BS; MA TC, Columbia University, NY. She has had a variety of nursing experiences including assistant executive director and executive director of the Michigan Nurses Association from 1956-

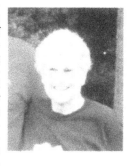

70. She joined the Veterans Administration in 1971, serving in five different states.

While active in MNA, she was appointed membership on the Michigan Governor's commission on the Status of Women under two administrations.

During the early days of certification, she became certified in Gerontological and Nursing Administration (ANA).

Married to Richard L. VerLee, she has

three step-children. She is a three time cancer survivor: breast cancer (both sides) and renal cell carcinoma. Other health problems are resolving thanks to the prayers of many people.

Retiring in 1990, she and Richard traveled to many states and foreign countries. Reading is an important hobby as well as church activities. They enjoy keeping up with family and friends by e-mail.

FRED VOCINO, Labor Relations Representative, joined the MNA staff in 1991. Representing RNs in MNA's larger Staff Councils, he assists in contract negotiations and administration, and often serves as MNA's spokesperson during negotiations and at grievance appeals. His assignments have included Staff Councils at the University of Michigan, Borgess Medical Center, Sparrow Hospital, and several other public and private employers. In addition, Fred periodically assists in the Association's organizing efforts. Peers throughout the state consider him an authority on interest-based bargaining and systematic approaches to union-management cooperation programs.

Fred's work on behalf of working people crosses over to involvement in the broad labor community and political action. Prior to coming to MNA, he served for 15 years as an elected officer for a UAW local at Wayne State University. Fred holds a Bachelor of Fine Arts degree from Wayne State University.

KIM SUSAN WALKER, born Feb. 10, 1957. She was influenced to become a nurse by a family friend, Ida Sillanpao, who was an RN. She gave Kim a nurse's cap when she was a little girl to play "nurse," and she still has the cap. Her father also encouraged her nursing career.

Attended Shapero School of Practical Nursing, Sinai Hospital, Detroit, MI; Troy State University, ASN, 1993 and BSN in 1997.

Assignments as US Army LPN, Honolulu, HI, Tripler Army Medical Center; Jackson Hospital, Montgomery, AL (Med/Surg) Central Alabama Home Health; Drug Research and Analysis, Montgomery, AL; Baptist Medical Center (ER) Montgomery, AL.

Awards: Charles L. Silcox Award for Excellence (Troy State University), Gamma Beta Phi Honor Society (Troy State University). Member of ANA, MNA and ONS.

Married to Mark, a paramedic, and they have daughters, Sidney Aiken (10) and Olivia Yang-Joy Mills (2). Currently, Kim is doing research at MSU (Family Care Studies) and Sparrow Health Systems (Medical Oncology).

JOAN WARNER, born May 5, 1955, Alpena, MI, and wanted to be a nurse from early childhood. Educated at Oakland Community Hospital as LPN in 1978 and New York University Regents Program in 1988 with associate degree in nursing.

She started working in Med/Surg for 12 years, ICU for five years, a step-down unit for five years, recovery for five years and is now a circle nurse in OR in a community hospital.

Awarded Advanced Cardiac Life Support, she is a basic life support instructor. Joan is a member of MNA, delegate to MNA convention for three years, member at large to Chapter 4, and she is also a member of the Order of the Eastern Star.

Joan and Larry have a daughter, Paula.

SUZANNE M. WEATHERS, BSN, MSN, born in Detroit, MI. Earned her BSN from Wayne State University and MSN from Oakland University. In addition to MNA, she has memberships in MONE, MLN and Sigma Theta Tau. She is the mother of three sons and is currently nursing program coordinator for Wayne County Community College District.

KATHY WEBER, born in Owosso, MI and aspired to nursing at an early age when she read the Clara Barton nurses series. In high school she volunteered as a candy striper at a nearby hospital. She received her diploma in nursing in 1972 after graduation from Hurley Hospital School of Nursing in Flint, MI.

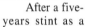

After a five-years stint as a public health nurse, Kathy began her hospital nursing career in 1978 at Lapeer County General Hospital (now Lapeer Regional Hospital), where she has spent the last 17 years in surgical services/endoscopy.

She has been an active member of the Lapeer RN Staff Council, MNA Bay Central Chapter, and the Michigan Chapter of Gastroenterolgy Nurses Association.

When not involved in professional activities, Kathy could be found vacationing to visit children and grandchildren or serving her church family at Grace Episcopal Church in Lapeer.

BARBARA WEIR, RN, born Oct. 4, 1932 in Jackson, MI at Mercy Hospital, the hospital at which she would graduate from 21 years later and become a registered nurse. Her mother being a registered nurse, she always had an inclination toward the medical profession.

She always appreciated the value of continuing education but decided to obtain formal education at Western University and received her BS in health administration in 1980 and her MS in public administration/health administration in 1986.

Her nursing experiences cover

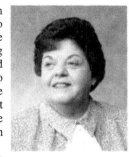

everything from general float to DON in the hospital setting until 1975 and then transferred to home care, she retired in 1997 at which time she opened a kitchen shop.

She has been a member of MNA for many years and held offices in both the state and county level and continues to be active in her retirement.

DIANE LARMOR WELKER graduated from Hurley School of Nursing in 1983. She worked as a staff nurse on the oncology unit at Hurley Medical Center while obtaining further education. She completed her BSN at the University of Michigan in Flint in 1987 and her master's in Oncology Nursing at Rush University in Chicago, IL in 1989.

Diane worked as an Oncology CNS for seven years, and an oncology nurse manager for four years before obtaining her Adult Nurse Practitioner Certification from Eastern Michigan University in 2001.

She wrote a booklet that was published worldwide through Sims Deltec titled *"Troubleshooting Vascular Access Devices."* The first edition was published in 1993 and the second edition will be out in 2004. She is currently employed at Hurley Medical Center as a coordinator for the Palliative Care Consultative Service. She and her husband Randy live in Lapeer with their two beautiful daughters, Courtney and Mackenzie, who are nurse wanna be's.

MONA LOUISE WHITE, born in Michigan and became interested in nursing when she was a young child and diagnosed with chronic asthma. She received an associate degree in nursing from Delta College in 1971 and worked in Intensive Care and Coronary Care before moving to Occupational Nursing. After rearing two sons with her husband Ken, she decided to pursue more education, receiving a BSN from Saginaw Valley State University in 1990 and a master of science of nursing in parenting and families from Wayne State University in 1993. She worked as a nurse educator teaching a variety of topics.

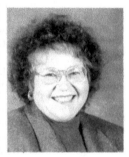

She received many honors during her career. She received the Michigan Outstanding Educator of the Year Award in 1997 and the Michigan Nurses Association

Excellence in Community and Child Nursing Award in 1998. She was the recipient of The YMCA Woman of the Millennium 2000. She was in *Who's Who in College Teachers* and a recipient of Robert Wood Johnson Foundation Grant to study End-Of-Life Nursing Education.

She was a member of Sigma Theta Tau, International Honor Society of Nursing, the American Nurses Association where she served as a Delegate to the ANA Convention. She was a member of the National League, chairing the task group on the Recruitment and Retention of Nursing Students. This work resulted in a Monograph published by the NLN.

She demonstrated leadership, serving on many committees. She was a member of the MNA Board of Directors representing the Bay Central Chapter. She also was president, vice-president and secretary of that chapter. She chaired the Transcultural Nursing Council for MNA and was a member of the MNA Task Force to Board of Nursing and the secretary MNA/MLN Task Force on Recruitment into Nursing. She also was the MNA Board Representative to COMON serving as vice-president. She represented her chapter on the Nurse Practice Council and chaired the Nominations Committee. She also served on the Reference Committee and the Nurses Impact Planning Committee.

She was a member of the National Nurse Practitioner Association and the Mid Michigan Advanced Practice Nurses Network.

She was actively involved in her community serving as chair of the Board of Directors of the Bay Area Women's Center and mentor for survivors of domestic violence and sexual assault. She earned credentials as a sexual assault nurse examiner. She was the nursing consultant for Freeland School District Human Sexuality Advisory, and was a frequent presenter on human sexuality issues, death and dying, positive thinking and motivation.

She was a frequent test item writer and consultant for National League for Nursing, Regents College New York, and National Council of State Boards of Nursing. She was also the author Critical Thinking Questions and Case Studies for a Maternal Child text and web site.

She traveled to China and Russia as ambassador through the American Nurses' Association to meet nursing colleagues face-to-face to discuss common nursing problems, compare recent research findings and evaluate areas for further collaboration. Mona died in a boating accident Memorial Day weekend, 2004.

IRENE A. WHITNEY, RN, Staff RN, born in Grand Rapids, MI and has a diploma in nursing. She has worked at Kent County Health Dept., St. Mary's Hospital and Visiting Nurses Service in Grand Rapids, MI.

Currently, she is staff position in Home Care at VNS.

Irene is a life member of Mercy Central School of Nursing Alumnae and a member of MNA. Her accomplishments are good marriage and relationships, family, friends, many lifelong friendships and patients. She has three grown children.

CAROL MERIAM WILLIAMS, Staff Nurse, Head Nurse, born Dec. 22, 1944 in Lakewood, OH. Graduated from University of Michigan with BSN in 1966 and MS in nursing health service administration in 1982 from UM.

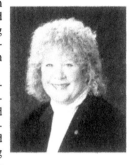

Carol is certified in Staff Development and Continuing Education; awarded Outstanding Nurse in Staff Development/Continuing Education by MNA in 1998 and Outstanding Nurse Educator from Chapter 8 of MNA in 2001; also, Chapter 8, MNA, delegate and CE Provider Unit representative.

Previously staff nurse, assistant head nurse, head nurse in Maternal Child Nurseries, assistant director of pediatric nursing, nursing information coordinator in Information Technology Dept., educational nurse specialist at UM and currently the nurse planner for the CE Provider Unit at UM Health System.

Her husband is retired from property management; they have two grown daughters, one owns a property management business and the other is an attorney, and three wonderful grandsons.

MARY MELISSA WILLIAMS, LPN, BSN, born April 15, 1954 in Ann Arbor, MI. She decided to become a nurse while taking care of a great aunt who became ill in her 80s and who had been a healthy independent until then. She earned her LPN in 1978, WCC; AD in 1984, WCC; and BSN at University of Michigan.

Member of MNA, ANA; also served on Perinatal Education Committee and Professional Practice Council at UMMC.

Mary worked in Med/Surg, psych, maternal child healthcare at UM for 25 years. In 1995 she left the hospital and went to work with Briarwood Medical Group, Internal Medicine, OB/GYN, case management, OB patient and staff education.

Married, she has three children, Megan, Brittney and Kaitlyn, ages 23, 19 and 17.

MICHAEL L. WILLIAMS, MSN, RN, CCRN, was born March 1, 1960 in Tecumseh, MI. He graduated from Michigan State University with a BS in medical technology,

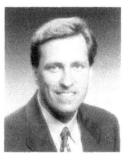

Lansing Community College (LCC) with an ADN in 1984 and his MSN from Grand Valley State University (GVSU) in 1989.

Michael began working as a graduate nurse in the Medical-Respiratory ICU of Ingham Medical Center. In 1990, Michael began working at the UM Hospitals and received the Excellence in Clinical Practice-CNS award in 1995. In 2002, Mr. Williams received a Distinguished Alumni Award from both Kirhkof School of Nursing, GVSU and from LCC, Lansing, MI, and Lifetime Membership Award from the American Association of Critical-Care Nurses (AACN). Michael is a member of Sigma Theta Tau International Honor Society, Michigan Nurses Association, the American Assembly for Men in Nursing, and AACN for which he served as the first male president from 2001-2002.

REGINA SALLEE WILLIAMS, a native of Sandusky, OH cannot remember when she did not have a love of learning and a particular interest in nursing. Admitted to Mount Carmel School of Nursing in Columbus, OH, she became one of the first four African American students to graduate

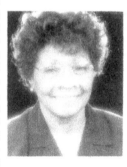

from the school in 1952. She received a BS from Ohio State University in 1955, a MS in nursing from Wayne State University and a PhD from the University of Michigan.

She taught nursing at Grant Hospital School of Nursing, Columbus, OH, 1958-65; at Mercy School of Nursing of Detroit, 1966-73; and at Wayne State University, College of Nursing, 1977-90. She was Interim Assistant Dean when she left Wayne State to accept an appointment as Head of the Department of Nursing at Eastern Michigan University in Ypsilanti, MI. She retired from Eastern Michigan University in August 2001.

In 1983, she was the first African-American to be elected president of Michigan Nurses Association. She was president of Michigan Association of Colleges of Nursing Dean's group from 1996-98. She was appointed to the State Board of Nursing where she served from 1987-96 and was chair of the board the last two years of her tenure.

She has received numerous awards and

certificates for meritorious service. Among these are awards from Detroit Black Nurses Association, the Michigan Nurses Association, Chi Eta Phi Nursing Sorority and Wayne State Chapter, Sigma Theta Tau International. She has been honored by proclamations and letters of commendation from the Honorable John Engler, Governor of Michigan; the Honorable Jackie Vaughn, Michigan Senator; the Michigan Senate; the Ohio Senate; and the Detroit City Council. She is an elected Fellow of the Nightingale Society and of the American Academy of Nursing. In 1996, Mount Carmel College of Nursing named her its Distinguished Alumni.

Although retired she remains active in nursing as a consultant, through attendance at conferences and by serving on several Advisory Boards. She is a member of Gesu Catholic Church in Detroit. She is married to Robert, a retired public school teacher. They have two adult children, Regina Mary of Washington, DC, and Peter Mark of Detroit.

LISA WOJNO, RN, Clinical Nurse II, born May 31, 1972 in Warren, MI. She possessed a passion for helping people and decided to become a nurse when touring NICU as a child. She graduated cum laude from Oakland University with a BSN and was a member of the Golden Key National Honor Society.

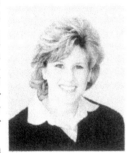

She began her career at Royal Oak Beaumont Hospital in Oncology and the Surgical ICU. She worked five years as a Clinical Nurse II in Labor and Delivery and several years in the EC as an insurance authorizer.

Concerned about health care and the future of nursing she decided to seek elective office. In 2002, Lisa was elected to the Michigan House of Representatives to serve the 28th District of Warren and Center Line. She is a member of the Health Policy Committee and is one of three RN's in the State Legislature. She is married to Paul and they have three children: Kennedy, Bradley and Audrey.

PAMELA D. WOJTOWICZ, born in Mt. Clemens, MI, is the executive assistant to the executive director of MNA. She has worked in the administrative field for over 30 years and enjoys the variety that a job of this type entails. She joined the staff of MNA in February 1999 and has worked for three executive directors of the association during that time. She has many responsibilities within her job, but assisting the executive director and the board of directors remain her most important priorities.

She is married and lives in Holt, MI. She has two children and three grandchildren. She is an avid mystery reader and spends much of her spare time reading, traveling and enjoying her family.

BARBARA WOOLARD, born July 16, 1957, Flint, MI. She started her career as a LPN and returned to school after 15 years for associate degree in nursing from Mott Community College.

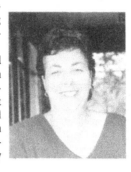

She worked as a staff nurse in ICU and Radiology for 10 years at Lapeer Regional Hospital, then Stress Lab at Regional Cardiology Association.

Barbara is past head of 1st strike at Lapeer Regional Hospital over staffing issues; assisted in developing staff nurse input in staffing issues; president of Lapeer MNA Union; and ACLS.

She and her husband have three boys who are active in the Boy Scouts of America and they are members of Free Methodist Church.

ALYSON WOLVIN, RN, born in Jackson, MI, wanted to be a RN for as long as she can remember. Her mother, also a RN, was her role model. She graduated from Jackson Community College with an associates degree in nursing. Currently she is working on a BA in labor studies through the National Labor College.

She brings 11 years of experience as a staff nurse in the Jackson area, including four years at Doctor's Hospital where she served on the Organizing Committee that was successful in their campaign to organize the hospital's RNs with the Michigan Nurses Association.

She joined the MNA staff in November 1998. As a labor organizer, she works with nurses across the state, interested in organizing a union in their healthcare facility. She is responsible for organizing campaigns from the first contact, through building and training the organizing committees, to the signing of a contract. She provides internal organizing education within existing MNA bargaining units, and works with other MNA organizers to develop customized campaign and training materials.

She is the mother of two beautiful children who are the joy of her life. Along with working to carry out the mission of MNA, she is blessed by spending time with her family and friends.

HEATHER F. WORDEN, BSN, RN. Her interest in nursing began in 1998 when she was a senior in high school searching for the perfect career. Much prayer, research, and guidance from a close friend (a RN), led Heather to the profession in which she now practices as a BSN, RN. She has no regrets and feels that God always had it in His plan for her to be a nurse.

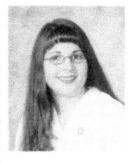

Heather practices on a medical cardiology unit. She is a member of Sigma Theta Tau International and is involved with MNA's Bay Central Chapter via the Congress on Nursing Practice. She is a graduate of Saginaw Valley State University's nursing program and hopes to continue her education and become involved in research, teaching, and policy-making. Heather feels that nurses are uniquely equipped to be advocates, health educators, coordinators of effective care, and partners in the provision of comfort. With the grace of God, she hopes to be a nurse that carries out all of these functions.

Heather is the youngest of four children and has extremely supportive parents and friends.

CHRISTINA MICHELLE WRAY, RN, BSN, Public Health Nurse, born May 31, 1979, Lansing, MI. Earned her associate in arts in education, associate in science and BS, all from Ferris State University and started the Graduate Program at Grand Valley State University in January 2004.

In August 2003 she started working for Kent County Public Health Dept. in Community Nursing Division with Maternal and Infant Support Services, helping pregnant young women and new moms to build better relationships with children and enhance growth and development.

She was awarded the Lona Lewis Scholarship; Dr. Hilda Richards Career Mobility Recipient and 2002 Faculty Award for Nursing Mentor.

Other activities include West Michigan Kalamazoo, Muskegon BNA, Big Brother/Big Sisters, Ferris Student Nurse Association. She served as student representative on National Black Nurse Association and studied transcultural nursing abroad in Finland in 2003.

Single, she has loving parents, sister and two-month-old nephew (was at the delivery of his birth).

CORA YEE, RN, BSN, Clinical Care Coordinator, born June 6, 1946, Bauan, Batangas, Philippines. Earned her BSN at University of St. Tomas, Manila, Philippines.

Awards include Excellence in Nursing, UM, 1992 and Nurse of Year in 2000, Hope Clinic. She is member of AAACN, UST

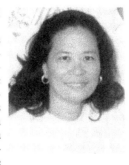

Nurses Alumni Association.

She has worked in ambulatory care, rheumatology clinic and UM hospitals. Her 14 years working at Burn Center made her a stronger and fulfilled person. She built friendships there that will last a lifetime. She is now in her 27th year of nursing at Michigan and proud of it.

Married to Edward who is a respiratory therapist at Ann Arbor VA Hospital. Their daughter Kimberly is a second year medical resident at the UM, and son Christopher is a senior and a captain of men's track team at UM.

MARICHAD YOUNG, Clinical Nurse I, born in December 1975 in Baton Rouge, LA. She got her associates degree from Washtenaw Community College, MS, bachelor's degree in science of nursing from University of Michigan.

Awards include university honors and Angell Scholar from UM. She is a member of Sigma Theta Tau Nursing Honor Society and volunteers for various fundraisers for burn patients.

She is working as a nurse at the Trauma Burn Center, University of Michigan Hospital and plans on returning to graduate school next year. She is the mother of two children.

FRANCES M. ZAJAC, Nurse Practitioner, born July 6, 1947. Earned her BSN at UM in 1969 and MSN at Wayne State Clinic in 1976. She received the Michigan Advanced Practice Nurse of the Year in 1989.

Active in Council of Nurses in Advanced Practice, Project MUSCLE, started MNA's legislative action on initial task force. Practice with Henry L. Green, MD, 1976-2002 and presented NP Symposiums Preceptor for MSN students.

Married to Michael, an attorney at BC/BS of Michigan and they have three boys: Michael (born 1982), Thomas (born 1985)

and William (born 1989). Currently, she is ANP, Cardiovascular Services at Mt. Clemens Hospital.

CAROL ZAWODNY, RN, born Aug. 18, 1949, Howell, MI and attended UM, Oakland Community College with an associate degree from Mott Community College. A past delegate her accomplishments are BLS, ACLS, Relief Charge Nurse.

Has worked on general medical floor, surgical, ICU, telemetry, endoscopy, recovery room and outpatient. Recently she returned to work after being off on a surgical leave. She will never forget what special people she works with – the many cards, phone calls and gifts gave her much needed encouragement to return to work.

Married 29 years to Frank with two sons, Frank and Dylan, and grandchildren, Ryan and Alexis. They have a 80 acre beef and crop farm and enjoy boating in their spare time. Currently Carol is a full time RN in the Surgery/Outpatient area

KAREN R. ATWELL-ZBICIAK, RN, BSN, Nurse Educator, Staff Nurse, born May 29, 1950 in Flint, MI. In 1971 the choices for women were teacher, nurse, secretary. She wanted to go away to school, but financially could not afford the universities. St. Joseph School of nursing was in town, affordable and they required the students to

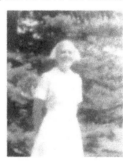

live in the dorm. When she went to check it out she remembers seeing all the smiling students and applied.

Received her diploma in 1971 from St. Joseph School and her BSN from UM in Flint, MI, in 1991. She loves nursing because of the wide variety of avenues you can take with it.

She has worked in Peds, Med-Surg, ICU, Post-Partum, Nursery, Hospice, Physician Office, Hospital Nurse Education, Col-

lege, and parish nurse at St. John the Evangelist Catholic Church in Davison, MI. She is a member of ANA, MNA, Bay Central. Currently she is working part-time, Faculty Mott Community College and Faculty Baker College, Casual Genesys Health System, Pediatrics, Women Surgery.

Married 23 years, she has one daughter, two step-sons and daughters-in-laws.

DILLIE M. ZILAFRO was born July 17, 1942 in Detroit, MI. She received her AD in Nursing from Henry Ford Comm. College, BSN from the U. of Michigan, and MSN with Nurse Practitioner from Indiana U.

She worked on the staff of Mt. Carmel (Hospital) for 10 years; private duty at Henry Ford Hospital; Munson Hospital Traverse for 17 years; teaching staff, Northwestern Michigan College Nursing Dept. for 12 years; Director and Nurse Practitioner for Community Health Clinic, Traverse City, for four years; Nurse Practitioner West Michigan Infertility for four years; and for the past seven years has been in private practice as a Nurse Practitioner for her business, Health Care For Today.

She is married and has two children and five grandchildren.

DEBBIE ZINGER, RN, CRRN, Staff Nurse, born Sept. 9, 1957, Grand Rapids, MI. Influenced by her grandmother who was born in 1900 and encouraged her to go into nursing. Her family profession is teaching and Debbie broke the mold when she went into nursing. She is a graduate of GRJC, associate degree in nursing in 1978; CRRN certified in 1998; and currently pursuing to continue education at GVSU for BSN.

She has worked in doctor's office, was a personal scrub nurse for two ophthalmologists for three years, did in-home health care for seven years, insurance rehab nurse for three years, church nurse for one year and visiting nurse for 11 years. Currently she is staff nurse with Visiting Nurses Services, SW Michigan.

Married 25 years to Steve, they have two children, Luke and Melanie, both attend Western Michigan University.

CHERYL A. CARLEVATO, Psychiatric Nurse Specialist, was born in Kalamazoo, MI. She received her AAS in Nursing from Delta College University Center Michigan. Her career began after high school graduation as a nurses aide, and she fell in love in nursing.

She worked for 16 years at Saginaw General Hospital, 10 years in Long Term Care as the Primary Coordinator and Instructor, CENA Training Program, Infection Control, Staff Development, Asst. DON and DON. Today she works for the Saginaw County Community Mental Health Authority, doing pre-admission screening and annual resident reviews for OBRA Geriatric Assessments.

She is a member of the Michigan Activity Therapists Conference Committee. Cheryl has been married (to the same man) for 26 years and has three terrific, nearly adult children.

PAMELA J. CHAPMAN was born April 5, 1952 in Detroit, MI. She feels she was born to be a nurse. She began her career as a licensed practical nurse in 1971.

In 1986 she received an ADN from Southwestern Michigan College. She joined the MNA in 1987. She has served the MNA in many capacities. She presently serves as president for MNA Chapter 5. She received her BSN in 2000 from FSU.

Pam has taken advantage of the many opportunities that nursing has to offer. She has practiced nursing across the life span. She presently practices as a care manager, performing utilization reviews and discharge planning.

Pam has a loving and supportive husband, two children and two grandchildren. Second to Christ, her family is the center of her life and joy. She enjoys humor and laughter; she is a professional clown.

She worships at the Mount Zion Baptist Church.

MARGUERITE (ROBERTSON) CURTIS, MSN, PhD, RN, CNP, was born Oct. 20, 1938 in Detroit, MI. She is a Leadership Saginaw graduate (1991); member of the National Association of Career Women; and was Saginaw Chapter Career Women of the Year (1998).

She established Professional Nursing Associates - Healthcare of Women in Saginaw (an independent nursing practice); served as President, Saginaw Bay District Nurses (1980s), which is now the AKA Bay Central Chapter, MNA. She was a member of the MNA Membership Marketing Committee (1980s).

Now semi-retired, Marguerite has lived in Hemlock, MI since 1977. She is married to James E. Curtis, Sr. and has four children: James E. Curtis, Jr., Margaret Laski, Jeanne Hanewich, and Catherine Hoeppner, and 12 grandchildren.

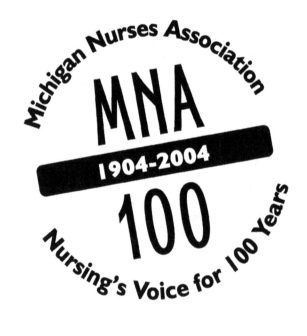

Printed in the USA
CPSIA information can be obtained
at www.ICGtesting.com
JSHW060045150824
68134JS00031B/2641